Also by Deirdre Imus

Green This! Volume 1: Greening Your Cleaning

The Imus Ranch: Cooking for Kids and Cowboys

growing up green:

baby and childcare

volume two in the bestselling green this! series

deirdre imus

simon & schuster paperbacks

new york london toronto sydney

Simon & Schuster
1230 Avenue of the Americas
New York, NY 10020

Copyright © by Git'R Green, Inc.

First Simon & Schuster trade paperback edition April 2008

SIMON & SCHUSTER and colophon
are registered trademarks of Simon & Schuster, Inc.

For information about special discounts for bulk purchases,
please contact Simon & Schuster Special Sales at 1-800-456-6798
or business@simonandschuster.com

**This book was printed using postconsumer recycled chlorine-free paper
and environmentally friendly inks.**

Designed by Davina Mock

Manufactured in the United States of America

10   9   8   7   6   5   4   3   2   1

Library of Congress Cataloging-in-Publication Data
Imus, Deirdre.
Growing up green : baby and child care / Deirdre Imus.
p. cm. — (Green this! ; v. 2)
Include bibliographical reference and index.
1. Green movement. 2. Environmentalism. 3. Pregnancy—Environmental aspects.
4. Infants—Care—Environmental aspects. I. Title.
GE195.I49 2008
649'.1—dc22
2007040911
ISBN-13: 978-1-4165-4124-0
ISBN-10:   1-4165-4124-1

For the loves of my life
Don and Wyatt Imus

acknowledgments

Thank you to Laura Moser, my writer. You were a joy to work with.

Thanks to my editor, Amanda Murray, for all your support. Special thanks to Bobbie Manning.

Again, I adore and thank my agent, Esther Newberg.

Thanks to David Rosenthal.

A special thank you to everyone at the Deirdre Imus Environmental Center for Pediatric Oncology at Hackensack University Medical Center: Bonnie Eskenazi, LaRae Muse, Erin Ihde, Mark Blaire, Jim Ronchi and David Marks for all your support and help.

Thank you as well to all the doctors, specialists and scientists for taking the time to talk with me and share valuable information that will help parents to better nurture and care for their children.

I thank Don, Wyatt, and Virgil for their endless love, humor and support.

contents

one: the wake-up call

1. A Letter to Parents   3

2. The Role of the Environment in Our Children's Health   9
   Environmental Triggers   11
   Toxic Triggers and Childhood Cancer   13
   Prevention Is the Best Cure   15

two: from utero to university

3. Preparing for Pregnancy   19
   Greening Your Thinking   19
   Greening Your Home   29

4.. Eating Right for Two   53
   The ABCs of Organic Eating   57
   Fish During Pregnancy: The Mercury Problem   59
   Spotlight On: Fetal Alcohol Spectrum Disorders   62

5. PREGNANCY AND BIRTH   66
        The Healthiest Pregnancy Possible?   66
        Some Simple Guidelines   70
        Choosing the Right Hospital   76

6. DEVELOPING YOUR BABY'S PALATE   78
        Nursing   82
        Better Bottles   85
        Organic Baby Food   87
        Got Milk?   89
        A Word on Microwaves   92
        Blue Moon Treats   94

7. INFANCY AND EARLY CHILDHOOD   96
        Playtime: Rethinking Your Toy Philosophy   97
        Bathing Your Baby   108
        Relaxation Techniques   111
        Teething Tools   112
        The Diaper Dilemma   113
        Sun Protection   115
        The Pet Question   116

8. "GREEN" PEDIATRICS   120
        *Vaccinations: Medicine's Greatest Achievement or Too Much
            of a Good Thing?*   122
        Spotlight On: *Autism and Autism Spectrum Disorders*   143
        The Rise of Childhood Allergies   148
        Antibiotics Overload   152
        Spotlight On: *Juvenile Rheumatoid Arthritis*   154
        Green Cures   156

9. OFF TO SCHOOL   167

Potential School Hazards   167

The School-Day Diet   171

Spotlight On: *Childhood Obesity and Diabetes*   174

Exercise: *The Most Essential Homework of All*   177

Spotlight On: *Attention Deficit/*
        Hyperactivity Disorder   180

The Happy Pill: Why Are We Overmedicating
        Our Kids?   183

Treating Head Lice   189

Pesticides on Playing Fields   192

Spotlight On: *Asthma*   193

Green School Gear   195

Greening Your After-School Activities   197

10. ADOLESCENCE AND BEYOND   199

Diet and Lifestyle   200

The Power of Fitness   202

Stress and Self-Reliance   203

Spotlight On: *Precocious Puberty*   206

Toxic Temptations   207

Future Preparations   210

11. BEYOND THE HOME: COMMUNITY ACTIVISM AND OUTREACH   212

Advocate for Organic Foods   213

Campaign for Cleaner Air   213

Carpool   214

Green the Cleaning at Your Children's School   214

Begin a Recycling Program   214

Advocate for Green Urban Development   215

Start a Local Community Garden or Farmer's Market   216
Support Child-Friendly Legislation   216

three: resources
Food   221
Recommended Reading   246
Buying Green: A Web Reference Guide   256
Important Legislation   262
Studies on Children's Health   265
Glossary of Environmental Health Terms   273
Biographies of Medical Experts   281

one:
the wake-up call

Chapter 1

A Letter to Parents

Half a century ago, most parents had a pretty good sense of their responsibilities toward their children: to provide them with food, clothing, shelter, an education, and, of course, love. Like parents throughout history, they did whatever was in their power to keep their children safe, to protect them from harm.

But what does it mean today, to "keep our children safe"? In recent years, the job of raising—and protecting—our children seems to have become a lot more complicated. Our lifestyles have undergone radical changes over the past few decades, and so has the environment we live in.

As a culture, we seem to be in constant motion. We work more, and sleep less, than ever before. Instead of making time for a good old-fashioned sit-down dinner at home, we opt for the drive-in window of the nearest fast-food restaurant. We live off processed foods loaded with sugars, synthetic additives, and trans fats. We skip our morning walk and instead spend hours of every day locked inside our cars or plugged into various electronic devices.

And perhaps most significantly, harmful toxins have become more and more present in our environment. Every week, more chemicals are introduced into our environment, often without first being tested for safety on humans, much less safety on children. These toxins pervade every aspect of our lives: the air we breathe, the water we drink, even the clothes we wear. We spray our lawns with pesticides, and eat fish contaminated with mercury, and drink milk pumped up with hormones. We sleep on mattresses treated with bioaccumulative flame retardants and scrub our kitchens—and our faces—with irritating chemicals. We're inundating ourselves with toxins twenty-four hours a day, seven days a week, and most of the time we don't even know it!

So what, you might be asking, does any of this have to do with raising a child?

The answer is absolutely everything. Over the past thirty years, these changes in our lifestyle, diet, and environment have taken a dramatic—and tragic—toll on our children's health. We're seeing epidemic levels of diabetes and obesity. Pediatric cancers have risen steadily at a rate of 1 percent annually over the last twenty years. A poor diet and lack of exercise have contributed to an epidemic of childhood obesity, with one in six children in the United States between the ages of six and nineteen considered overweight. Asthma rates have increased tenfold over the last decade. Approximately one out of every six U.S. children has a developmental disability, including speech and language disorders, learning disabilities, and attention deficit/hyperactivity disorder (ADHD). Approximately 1 in 150 American children has an autism spectrum disorder (ASD).One out of every eight babies is born premature in this country, and the rate of premature births increased nearly 31 percent between 1981 and 2003. Rheumatoid arthritis has become the third-most-common childhood disease—among *infants*. Childhood allergies are at record levels.

If you're like me, you probably feel pretty horrified upon confronting these sobering facts for the first time. But I don't want this information to frighten or paralyze you. On the contrary: It should empower you to start asking some critical questions about what's causing this extraordinary increase in diseases over the last twenty-five years and what you as a parent can do to reverse these trends.

The World Health Organization estimates that we could prevent more than 80 percent of all chronic illnesses by improving our lifestyles in simple ways, like working to reduce our exposure to environmental pollutants and eating a healthier diet. Eighty percent! So why aren't we doing more to protect our children?

For a number of reasons, children are more adversely affected by exposure to environmental toxins than adults. Pound for pound of body weight, they breathe and eat more than we do. Their still-developing immune systems might mistakenly treat the toxins as naturally occurring enzymes or hormones. And because children are growing and developing so fast, dangerous cell mutations can multiply at a faster rate. Children are also less capable of detoxifying and excreting chemicals than adults. Their blood-brain barrier is still porous and allows more chemicals to reach their brains.

The environmental toxins most harmful to children include:

- Mercury (in vaccines, fish, dental amalgams, coal-burning emissions, incinerators, landfills)
- Toxic cleaning products
- PCBs (polychlorinated biphenyls)
- Lead
- Air pollutants such as dioxins, volatile organic compounds (VOCs), asbestos
- Environmental and/or tobacco smoke
- Pesticides sprayed in the home and on the lawn
- Pesticides used in lice shampoos

- Pesticides in food and water
- Drinking water contaminants
- Industrial emissions

Many children, particularly those in lower-income urban areas, face a number of these environmental insults on a regular basis, even daily. All I can say is no *wonder* their health is suffering. Their bodies are overloaded with toxins and deficient in the nutrients they need to develop properly. How could our kids *not* be chronically ill?

As parents, and as a society, we need to become more vigilant about shielding our children from these environmental insults. We're already way past the tipping point. We can—we *must*—band together to reverse these frightening trends in our children's health.

With that goal in mind, I've written this book for *you*—all the concerned parents (and future parents) out there who are ready to take charge of their children's health once and for all. *Greening Your Baby* is a chronological, stage-by-stage guide that will take you from the moment you first entertain the possibility of having a child all the way through the moment when you send that child off into the "real world," whether that means college or the workplace. Whatever your level of parenting experience, if you have one kid or nine, you can use the information in these pages to secure a better future for your children.

With the necessary tools, you *can* protect your children from environmental toxins. Throughout this book, I'll be examining how all sorts of different lifestyle choices—about nutrition, physical fitness, even vaccinations—may affect the development of your child. I've spoken to more than twenty of the most respected children's health experts in the country about the dangers toxins pose and the actions we can take to reduce kids' exposure to them.

Though I was interested in these issues long before I became a mother, the birth of my son, Wyatt, deepened my determination to clean up our toxic environment. I wanted to give my son the best possible start in life, and I knew that doing so meant reducing his exposure to toxins. How could I help Wyatt and millions of kids like him?

In 1998—the same year that I gave birth to Wyatt—my husband and I realized a longtime dream when we founded the Imus Ranch in Ribera, New Mexico. That summer, and every summer since, we invited children suffering from cancer and various life-threatening blood disorders, such as sickle cell, and children who have lost a brother or sister to sudden infant death syndrome, to experience life on our authentic 1880s-style working cattle ranch.

My experiences over the last decade at the ranch have strengthened my desire to leave our children, and their children, a cleaner world to inherit. We've now had more than seven hundred kids at the ranch, and I've learned a great deal from every single one of them. I like to think that this book reflects many of the lessons I've taken from my summers in New Mexico—and from every day of the year as a mother.

To me, it all boils down to knowing the right questions to ask and the choices that are available to you. Awareness is the essential tool here. Only when we truly educate ourselves about the widespread threats to our children's health can we take steps to avoid and ultimately eliminate those threats. With that goal in mind, in 2001, I founded the Deirdre Imus Environmental Center for Pediatric Oncology at the Hackensack University Medical Center in Hackensack, New Jersey, to raise people's awareness of the environmental factors that contribute to childhood cancer and other serious childhood diseases. In our campaign to reduce kids' exposure to environmental toxins, we place a big emphasis on the dangers of cleaning chemicals and pesticides in schools and homes. We believe that if more parents spoke out about the irreparable harm these substances were doing to our children, people would no longer use them.

The time has come to raise our voices and demand some changes. If we continue bringing up our children in this toxic soup, their health problems will only worsen, and then what will we be left with as a society?

Throughout this book, I've tried to make my suggestions as accessible, realistic, and affordable as possible, since I'm the first to acknowledge that most parents have too much on their plates for any complicated life-turnaround scheme. Even if, like so many families today, you and your partner both have full-time jobs, I promise you that you *can* make these changes, without any trouble at all. I've always believed that the most significant transformations are the ones that occur slowly, sometimes without our even noticing.

As you read, I'd like you to revisit the question I introduced at the very beginning: What does it mean, these days, to keep your children safe, to protect them from harm? I'm talking about more than just buckling your seatbelt or locking the back door at bedtime. I'm talking about protecting your children's health over the long term.

Yes, the rules of the game have changed over the last few decades. But if there's one thing that parenthood teaches, it's adaptability. And there's no time like the present to put that skill to good use. We must adapt our lifestyles and diets to our children, before it's too late.

Chapter 2

The Role of the Environment
in Our Children's Health

W hen my son Wyatt was a baby, I began seeking more information about the off-the-charts increases in childhood health problems that we've see over the past two decades. Why are rates of certain diseases skyrocketing in our kids today? Does the environment play a role, or is the cause beyond our control, like a genetic mutation that makes us more vulnerable to disease?

I also wanted to find out what exactly a "genetic epidemic" is. The term, which frequently comes up in discussions of these disease increases, suggests that the population is experiencing widespread changes in DNA, simply in the normal course of evolution. But is that the root cause of all these childhood health problems? Do genes really change that fast?

When I asked the almost two dozen prominent doctors and researchers who I interviewed for this book to explain this concept to me, every single one of them told me point blank that *there is no such thing as a genetic epidemic.*

DNA simply cannot mutate fast enough to explain these sharp increases in childhood health problems. Dr. Phil Landrigan—the director of the Center for Children's Health and the Environment and the director of Environmental and Occupational Medicine at the Mount Sinai School of Medicine—told me that "genes do change over the millennia, but not in twenty years. I don't think any of these increases in diseases that we've been talking about are due to changes in children's genes. They're due to changes in the environment."

Dr. Frederica Perera, the director of Columbia University's Center for Children's Environmental Health and an internationally recognized leader in researching the environmental causes of cancer and developmental disorders, agreed. "Genes alone do not explain these increases," she said, "but they do play a role with the other factors. We have to think about all of these factors together." In other words, to understand the root cause of these childhood health problems, we must evaluate both genes and the environment, a category Dr. Landrigan defined in the broadest sense as "everything that's not your DNA": air pollution, nutrition, household products, and so on.

Dr. Joel Fuhrman, who specializes in preventing and reversing disease through holistic and dietary protocols, clarified the distinction between genetic and environmental contributors to disease. "We all have genetic differences," he told me. "There's great variability among the human genome, which makes some of us more susceptible to various environmental and toxic stresses than others. You may be more prone to heart disease, and another person may be more prone to a certain type of cancer. But it doesn't mean that without those environmental stresses they would've ever developed heart disease or cancer. It's not genetic in the sense that you can't do anything about it. It just means that under a certain set of environmental challenges, this body is more prone to develop certain weaknesses. Clearly, we're confusing genetic tendencies with the *cause* of these illnesses."

What these prominent researchers are saying—and what I've long believed—is that, when looking for the root cause of many diseases, you cannot consider genetics in a vacuum. You have to take the environment into account as well. Yes, our genes do play some role in our likelihood of developing these diseases, but that's just the beginning of the story. When you're seeing such out-of-control disease increases over such a short period of time, you have to look for another explanation. You have to ask what in the environment is causing such a high percentage of children to be vulnerable to these chronic illnesses.

And yet, for some reason, we devote the vast majority of our resources to making sense of genes and genetic diseases. When I asked Dr. Perera why we don't spend more money on researching environmental causes of disease instead, she said that it was because "measuring genes is precise, and you can do it beautifully. Measuring the environment isn't so pretty, so it doesn't always have that appeal. Genes are sexy and high technology, but you have to bring in the environment, too. You have to be studying both. When you are talking about prevention, it's the environmental factors you can change; the genes you can't change."

Precisely because we *can* change these environment factors, we must work harder at understanding how they affect our health. If as a society we paid more attention to the environmental causes of disease, we could do a better job of protecting our children.

Environmental Triggers

Researchers have linked environmental exposures to a jaw-dropping number of health problems: learning disabilities, hyperactivity, headaches, asthma, allergies, obesity, diabetes, autism, eye damage, pediatric cancer, and even rheumatoid arthritis. In its 2006 environmental health report, the Environmental Protection Agency (EPA) found that "avoidable environmental exposures" are responsible for as much as 24 percent of all global diseases and more than 33 percent of diseases in children under the age of five.

In an effort to improve children's health, the EPA has targeted a wide range of environmental threats, including indoor air quality (from building materials, toxins used in chemical cleaners); outdoor air pollution (from vehicle emissions, secondhand tobacco smoke, dry-cleaning fluids); pesticide use (both at home and in schools); and lead (in paint, drinking water, and toys). Scientists are beginning to link these and certain other common exposures—like heavy metals, pesticides, dioxins, flame retardants, and PCBs—to different health problems. And a number of recent studies reinforce links between prenatal exposure to environmental pollutants and childhood health problems. A 2004 Columbia study, for example, showed that babies born to nonsmoking women who lived within two miles of the World Trade Center weighed significantly less than full-term infants born in other areas of New York City. And a section of the Mothers and Children Study released by Columbia in 2006 established that prenatal exposure to polycyclic aromatic hydrocarbons (PAHs)—the byproduct of combustion from various sources—can adversely affect not only birthweight but neurocognitive ability during childhood. (For more studies on environmental pollutants and their impact on children's health, see page 265 in the resources section.)

Despite these significant research developments, we still have much, much more to learn about how environmental exposures affect human health. We're only just beginning to understand the extent to which everyday exposures, even at low levels, can leave us vulnerable to illness. To further complicate matters, more chemicals are being introduced into our environment every day, often without first being tested for safety. In fact, of the more than 82,000 chemicals present in our environment, only a tiny fraction of them have been thoroughly evaluated for their impact on human health, much less the health of children.

"We live in a chemical society," said Frances Beinecke, president of the Natural Resources Defense Council. "And we never have enough information on what the consequences of [82,000 chemicals] are. There's not enough testing ahead of time, or understanding about how those chemicals relate and react to one another, or how human exposure is affected."

And while we've done some research on the dangers these pollutants pose on an individual basis, we've yet to study the impact of all of these chemicals mixed together. And this, many researchers agree, is the crux of the issue: many of these illnesses are the result not of one single traumatic exposure, but of a combination of different, smaller exposures—a phenomenon sometimes referred to as the "synergistic effect."

Dr. Fuhrman described the source of the problem as a "whole constellation of different environmental insults." The effect of these toxins on a child's development, he said, is like "putting ingredients into a witch's cauldron. There are a lot of factors, a combination of environmental and nutritional challenges."

Given certain factors, he said, damage and disease are almost to be expected. Kids exposed to air pollution, for example, are more likely to have higher rates of asthma and allergies. Diet is another ingredient in the cauldron. "Kids' immune systems are suppressed—you can't have normal immune function on a diet with so much processed foods and animal products and a diet so low in fruits and vegetables and beans and nuts and seeds. You can't expose the body to so many immune-stimulating challenges and not expect to have some damages in the DNA."

Toxic Triggers and Childhood Cancer

I had many different motivations for founding my environmental center, but fighting childhood cancer was always at the top of my list. That's because, to me, the rising rates of childhood cancer are one of the most tragic outcomes of the toxic world we live in. Cancer—a disease that results from a complex interaction of genes and the environment—is now the leading cause of death by disease for U.S. children between the ages of one and nineteen. Between 1975 and 1998, rates of childhood cancer increased by approximately 21 percent. Certain other cancers—brain tumors, leukemia, acute lymphoblastic leukemia (ALL), and central nervous system malignancies—have grown at an even more rapid rate, about 30 percent over the last two decades. The National Cancer Institute estimates that these rates will continue to climb an additional 1 percent every year.

And why? What's causing these increases? "In my professional opinion, and according to the National Cancer Institute," said Dr. Devra Davis, the director of the Center for Environmental Oncology at the University of Pittsburgh Cancer Institute, "inherited risk accounts for fewer than one in ten cases of cancer. That means nine out of ten children who get cancer were born with perfectly healthy genes, but something has happened to them—sometimes prenatally—that gives them the disease.

"Only 10 percent of cancers are due to genes that we are born with," Dr. Davis told me, "which is a very small percentage." According to Robert N. Hoover of the National Cancer Institute, the remaining 80 to 90 percent are triggered by environmental exposures.

Susan Sencer, who directs the integrative cancer care program at Children's Hospitals and Clinics, Minneapolis–St. Paul, mentioned the "Knudson theory" of cancer causation. She explained: "This theory states that many cancers, and especially childhood cancers, take at least two hits—meaning you could be genetically predisposed but you must also have at least one other exposure to develop cancer. It's not enough to be born with the genes—you must also take at least one other hit. Of course, we don't know what the nature of the 'hit' is. It maybe viral, environmental, or something we currently don't understand at all."

The first hit, Dr. Sencer said, is your genes, but without the second hit from the environment, you probably won't get cancer. Dr. Davis offered a vivid analogy for the interplay between genes and the environment: "Your genes are the gun, but it's the environment that pulls the trigger. So that in nine out of ten cases, people don't get cancer because of the genes they got from their parents, but because of the environment in which they grew up. And that environment starts prenatally, of course."

Your job as parent is to monitor your children's environment so that this trigger never gets pulled.

Prevention Is the Best Cure

It's an old cliché that still rings true today: Prevention *is* the best cure for many of the problems that are threatening our children's futures. With some knowledge, and a few proactive measures, we can go a long way toward preventing our children from ever falling victim to these health problems. That's the goal of this book: to teach you, the parent, how to take control of your children's health.

Prevention should always be the focus of any health-care—and parenting—protocol. Minimizing the exposures that cause disease is much more effective, and less painful, than treating the disease after the fact.

Dr. Phil Landrigan offered a parallel to the cost of cleaning up environmental disasters. "It makes a lot more sense to go upstream and to stop the pollution at its source. It's always cheaper to prevent the pollution in the first place than to clean it up afterward. Look at the millions—the billions—of dollars that this country is spending on cleaning up Superfund sites and toxic waste sites. And that's all because five, ten, fifteen years ago, somebody carelessly threw a bunch of fifty-five gallon drums of some toxic chemical into a landfill and then forgot about it.

"Now, twenty years later, we're having to deal with the consequences. And it's horribly expensive. The cheapest approach would've been never to use the toxic chemical in the first place. The next cheapest would've been to deal with it right then and there, to find a safe way to deal with it. And the most expensive is to throw it over the back of a truck and leave it for the next generation."

We're doing the exact same thing with our kids—inundating them with toxic chemicals without any regard for the possible consequences of our actions or any real understanding of how these exposures might affect them five, ten, or fifteen years down the line. It's a perfect storm: nutritional deficiencies, environmental toxins, accelerated vaccine schedules, and the inability to detoxify all these toxins. Children's immature immune systems simply cannot cope with this toxic overload.

So wouldn't it make more sense to intervene before our kids ever get sick? That's precisely why I've written this book: to give you, the parents, the know-how to clean up your environment, so that you in turn can give your kids a healthier start in life.

two:
from utero to university

Chapter 3

Preparing for Pregnancy

As any parent can tell you, bringing a child into the world is a huge, huge deal. Until you have a child of your own, you can never fully anticipate how dramatically parenthood will transform your life. Once the baby arrives, your days will be hectic and your nights sleepless. If you're like most first-time parents, you'll be far too busy (and exhausted!) to overhaul your lifestyle in any significant way at this stage. Pregnancy can also be an overwhelming time, for first-time parents especially.

Greening Your Thinking

In an ideal world, you'll take the first steps toward greening your baby even earlier, prior to giving birth and even prior to getting pregnant. Don't wait until you're already a parent to start changing your habits. The lives we lead before conception—the foods we eat, the place we live, our exercise habits—also play a huge role in the health of our future children. About half of all pregnancies in this country are unplanned, and most women don't discover they're pregnant until the sixth week. In many cases, the baby's central nervous system is fully developed before a woman even knows she's pregnant. Therefore, you should take the first essential steps, like giving up cigarettes and alcohol, right away.

Dr. Kenneth Bock, the co-founder of the Rhinebeck Health Center and the author of *The Road to Immunity* and *Healing the New Childhood Epidemics: Autism, ADHD, Asthma and Allergies*, believes that reducing chemical exposures is key to optimizing the health of your baby. "And the first place I'd reduce exposures is in the preconception. If you can detoxify yourself—*yourselves*, actually [meaning both parents]—before you conceive, you have more of a chance of having healthier sperm, healthier eggs, a healthy environment in which those kids are going to be, hopefully, flourishing in utero."

So, while we often think that our child's life begins at the moment of conception or birth, parents-to-be—both mothers and fathers—need to take charge of their health *before* pregnancy. The sooner you detoxify, the better. But first, you need to familiarize yourself with some basic facts.

Getting Educated

And surely we are all out of the computation of our age, and every man is some months elder than he bethinks him; for we live, move, have a being, and are subject to the actions of the elements and the malice of diseases, in that other world, the truest Microcosm, the Womb of our Mother."
                              —Sir Thomas Browne, *Religio Medici* (1643)

The umbilical cord connects the mother to her baby, carrying blood and nutrients from the placenta to the child within the womb. Until just a few years ago, scientists believed that the placenta acted as a barrier between the developing baby and industrial pollutants in the environment. But a groundbreaking 2004 study by the Environmental Working Group (EWG) showed that the umbilical cord ferries "not only the building blocks of life, but also a steady stream of industrial chemicals, pollutants and pesticides that cross the placenta as readily as residues from cigarettes and alcohol." The EWG called this phenomenon the "human 'body burden'—the pollution in people that permeates everyone in the world, including babies in the womb."

From a cord-blood sample taken from ten randomly selected babies born in the United States in August and September of 2004, researchers found an astonishing 287 of the 413 industrial chemicals it tested for. These included perfluorochemicals, or PFCs (found in some stain and oil repellants); flame retardants used in the manufacturing of furniture foam, computers, televisions, and kids' furniture; metals (lead, mercury, arsenic, much of which enters the environment through burning coal, gasoline, and garbage), and chlorinated dioxins.

Tests show 287 industrial chemicals in 10 newborn babies
Pollutants include consumer product ingredients, banned industrial chemicals and pesticides, and waste byproducts

Sources and uses of chemicals in newborn blood	Chemical family name	Total number of chemicals found in 10 newborns (range in individual babies)
Common consumer product chemicals (and their breakdown products)		47 chemicals (23–38)
Pesticides, actively used in U.S.	Organochlorine pesticides (OCs)	7 chemicals (2–6)

Sources and uses of chemicals in newborn blood	Chemical family name	Total number of chemicals found in 10 newborns (range in individual babies
Stain and grease resistant coatings for food wrap, carpet, furniture	Perfluorochemicals (PFCs)	8 chemicals (4–8)
Fire retardants in TVs, computers, furniture	Polybrominated di-phenyl ethers (PBDEs)	32 chemicals (13–29)
Chemicals banned or severely resticted in the U.S. (and their breakdown products)		212 chemicals (111–185)
Pesticides, phased out of use in U.S.	Organochlorine pesticides (OCs)	14 chemicals (7–14)
Stain and grease resistant coatings for food wrap, carpet, furniture	Perfluorochemicals (PFCs)	1 chemicals (1–1)
Electrical insulators	Polychlorinated biphenyls (PCBs)	147 chemicals (65–134)
Broad use industrial chemicals–flame retardants, pesticides, electrical insultators	Polychlorinated naph-thalenes (PCNs)	50 chemicals (22–40)

Sources and uses of chemicals in newborn blood	Chemical family name	Total number of chemicals found in 10 newborns (range in individual babies
Waste byproducts		28 chemicals (6–21)
Garbage incineration and plastic production wastes	Polychlorinated and Polybrominated dibenzo dioxins and furans (PCDD/F and PBDD/F)	18 chemicals (5–13)
Car emissions and other fossil fuel combustion	Polynuclear aromatic hydrocarbons (PAHs)	10 chemicals (1–10)
Power plants (coal burning)	Methylmercury	1 chemicals (1–1).
All chemicals found		287 chemicals (154–231)

Source: Environmental Working Group analysis of tests of 10 umbilical cord blood samples conducted by AXYS Analytical Services (Sydney, BC) and Flett Research Ltd. (Winnipeg, MB).

Every single child tested was born with a wide range of pollutants, many of which have been banned for decades. Of the 287 chemicals found, well over half—180—are known or suspected carcinogens in humans or animals. At least 217 have been shown to be toxic to the brain and nervous system, while 208 have been linked to birth defects or abnormal development in animal tests.

The findings of this Body Burden study speak for themselves. They emphasize the urgent necessity for parents to clean themselves up *before* pregnancy, to reduce their future children's exposure to these dangerous chemicals well ahead of time. Because while scientists have yet to evaluate the impact of this toxic chemical cocktail on developing fetuses and very young children, they do know that toxic exposures in the womb or during infancy can have a much greater effect than the same exposures later in life, even if the prenatal exposures occur at much lower levels.

Laying the Groundwork

Mothers with health problems—particularly obesity, diabetes, and hypertension—are more likely to have children with health problems. Fathers' health can also play a crucial role in the outcome of a pregnancy. Though this subject hasn't yet received enough attention, we do know that fathers with certain industrial and agricultural occupations are more likely to have children with neurocognitive problems.

So from the very beginning, get your partner involved in the greening process. Give up smoking as a team, and take turns cooking healthier recipes. Pay a visit to your doctor together. Evaluate your health to determine the risk factors involved on both sides, and see what steps you can take to minimize these risks. Dr. Manny Alvarez, the chairman of the Department of Obstetrics and Gynecology and Reproductive Science at Hackensack University Medical Center, strongly recommends this step, which many future parents skip.

"The ideal thing," he said, would be to go to your doctor and say, "'Hi, this is my significant other. We're thinking of having a baby.' And this is *before* you get pregnant. I'd say, 'OK, significant other, let's have a conversation. Let's see what your history is, let's see what your partner's history is, let's see what the two of you need to do beforehand.' And then you go and you have your wonderful little time together, and you come back pregnant. For the most part, those precautions could eliminate a lot of stuff."

If you've decided the time is right to try having a baby, you can make all sorts of little adjustments to clean up your life:

- Avoid inoculations with thimerosal in them. Flu shots often contain thimerosal, so check with your doctor before getting one.

- Get into a habit of regular exercise, either on your own or with the support of your partner. Don't just exercise when you find out you're pregnant; make it an essential part of your day-to-day life. (If you start now, before you get pregnant, you'll want to continue.) Exercise is a great detoxifier, so don't be afraid to sweat! The fitter you are, the easier your pregnancy—and the healthier your baby—will be.

- Give up drinking alcohol and start drinking filtered water (at least eight eight-ounce glasses a day) instead.

- Stop taking birth-control pills at least three months before trying to conceive.

- Start taking a prenatal vitamin with folate. Taking folic acid during your childbearing years has been shown to reduce the rish of certain birth defects by as much as 75 percent. (For more on the benefits of a folate supplement during pregnancy, see page 56.)

- Last but not least: Clean up your diet! The presence, or absence, of essential vitamins and minerals in your body can play a huge role not only during your pregnancy, but in the months that precede it. If you have the proper nutritional reserves in your body *before* you get pregnant, you can start supplying your baby with the nutrients she needs right away, in the very first days of your pregnancy, well before your first visit to the obstetrician. And start drinking filtered water to flush out the toxins. For specific eating tips, see chapter 4.

And if you're over the age of thirty-five, you should talk to your doctor about any additional precautions you should take before trying to get pregnant. Every year, more and more U.S. women fall into this category: In 2003, the average age of a mother giving birth for the first time rose to a record high of 25.2, an increase of almost four years since 1970. Between 1991 and 2001 alone, the number of first births per one-thousand women aged thirty-five to thirty-nine increased by 36 percent, and by 70 percent among women aged forty to forty-four.

While I think it's great that women today are waiting longer to start their families, prospective mothers over age thirty-five need to take stock of the risks they face during pregnancy, like developing gestational diabetes or high blood pressure. They're also more likely to be overweight or have more preexisting medical conditions than younger mothers. According to the March of Dimes, older mothers also run a greater risk of having miscarriages, multiple births, or a baby with birth defects or genetic disorders. So if you're over thirty-five and thinking about getting pregnant, be all the more vigilant about cleaning up your life well ahead of time.

Treating Infertility

These days, just getting pregnant can present big challenges: An estimated 5 to 10 percent of American couples have some difficulty conceiving. While researchers don't yet know all the reasons for infertility, many believe that the prevalence of hormone mimics and endocrine disruptors in our environment might play a role. Exposure to these chemicals—which can be present in everything from toxic plastics and conventional laundry detergents to organophosphate pesticides—could disrupt the body's hormone signals that regulate reproduction and development, either by blocking, mimicking, or interfering with the action of hormones.

"If left to our own devices, our bodies are really pretty good about making checks and balances," said Dr. Mady Hornig, an associate professor of epidemiology at Columbia University. "But there are now so many factors in the environment that mimic our natural hormones, and there's only so much adaptation our body's metabolic machinery can provide." To maximize their fertility, couples should make an effort to reduce contact with any agents, like PCBs (see page 39) that might alter their hormones.

Parents-to-be should also start asking more questions about how fertility treatments work. The standard course of treatment at a fertility clinic—first hormone treatments; then, if necessary, in vitro fertilization (IVF) or intracytoplasmic sperm injection (ICSI)—has helped a great number of people get pregnant, but how safe are these treatments? How much do we even know about how fertility treatments work? I believe in being a fully informed consumer in every aspect of life, and fertility treatments should be no exception. If my eggs were being perserved in a Petri dish, I know that I'd make it a priority to ask my doctor for a complete list of the preservatives being used. Before putting any substance into my body, I always make sure that I'm comfortable with all the ingredients. And just how thoroughly have fertility clinics tested the long-term safety of the substance used to preserve eggs? Could any of the chemicals used in popular fertility treatments be causing DNA damage? These chemicals have to be doing *something* to the cells, but what exactly? What are the long-term physical and developmental effects of fertility treatments?

I'm not saying fertility treatments are bad or good; I'm just saying that we need to start asking these and other questions. We also need to start demanding answers. We need to be absolutely certain that the preservatives used in these procedures are as safe as possible—we need to demand *proof*.

While many couples see no alternative but to undergo fertility treatments, there are other avenues worth exploring. Not just detoxifying your body, which is obviously essential, but finding ways to reduce stress (see page 71). "I'm interested in the interactions between the brain and the hormonal and immune systems," Dr. Hornig told me. "The brain has a lot of components, and stress is a very biochemical process that affects hormones and immunity. Is there something about uncertainty and stress that reduces the probability of getting pregnant? I don't know how we could measure that, but that could be interesting. If we could look at various stress hormones in women trying to get pregnant, we might find that stress hormones reduce their ability to get pregnant."

Finding a "sense of community and belonging that is, unfortunately, so often lacking in urban settings is another really critical element," Dr. Hornig said.

So before going straight to the fertility clinic, explore other methods. In her classic book *Taking Charge of Your Fertility*, Toni Weschler introduces the principles of the fertility awareness method (FAM), which teaches women how to chart their own menstrual cycles, determine when they're ovulating, and boost their chances of conception without recourse to drugs. Weschler encourages women to spend more time outside during daylight hours, and to try traditional Chinese medicine practices like acupuncture, which has proved very helpful both in reducing stress and in resolving the hormonal imbalances that can lead to infertility.

After an ectopic pregnancy and two miscarriages in just two years, I felt doomed. No matter what I did, I simply couldn't have that baby my husband and I had dreamed about for so long. I was only twenty-eight years old—what was wrong with me? I considered IVF, but it was so expensive, and in any event getting pregnant didn't seem to be my problem—it was bringing the baby to term. So, at the recommendation of a friend, I started going to an acupuncturist in Chinatown twice a week. In addition to the acupuncture, she gave me herbs and taught me relaxation techniques. I'd tried everything else, so why not? To this day, I don't know if it was the acupuncture itself, or the herbs, or just the emotional support of my doctor, but fifteen months after I started my acupuncture treatments, I gave birth to a beautiful baby boy.

Carolyn M., Portland, OR

GREENING YOUR HOME

A green environment starts at home. For best results, I always recommend getting back to the basics. With just a few minor adjustments, you can go a long way toward protecting your family's health over the long run. The changes I'm proposing are as easy as they are essential.

There are many simple practices parents—and prospective parents—can adopt to minimize exposure to potentially harmful substances. I strongly recommend trying out some of the following suggestions today, before you get pregnant, so that your good habits will already be in place when your baby arrives. Whether you end up having children or not, you and everyone around you will benefit from these easy household improvements.

Greening Your Shopping

Every day, all of us make hundreds of little decisions about how and where to spend our money. But as consumers, we don't just control the products that come into our household. On a broader scale, we also control the products that land on the shelves of our supermarkets and stores. If enough of us band together and refuse to buy toxic foods and clothes and cleaning products, I can guarantee that the industry standards will change. The more that we demand safe green products, the more widely available—and more affordable—these products will become. It really is that simple. Everything starts with what you buy and bring into your home. "The more consumer demand for green products that you have," Frances Beinecke told me, "the more the market will develop products that are better for people's health. And parents are an incredibly strong source for that movement."

So, even before you get pregnant, I ask that you commit to just one small change in the supermarket aisle. Replace your toxic cleaning product with a nontoxic one, or your chemical toothpaste with a natural brand. The next time you're in the produce section, opt for the organic apple instead of the one that's been sprayed with toxic pesticides. Buy an inexpensive filter to remove pollutants from the water you drink. Buy only rechargeable batteries. Recycle grocery bags or start bringing your own reusable bags to the grocery store.

I promise you that these tiny changes will lead to bigger improvements in the long run, without overwhelming you along the way. Take responsibility for the world your future children will one day inherit. You can start the next time you go shopping. By making these informed choices, you won't just be improving your family's health. You'll also be making a powerful statement to corporate America and paving the way for other concerned parents in the future. The more of us who commit to purchasing nontoxic consumer goods and reducing waste, the more widely available these products will become. So the next time you walk into your local supermarket or department store, remember that *you're* the one in control. Use your power responsibly.

Greening Your Cleaning

A truly healthy, toxin-free environment starts at home. Unfortunately, many ordinary household cleaners—toilet cleaners, window cleaners, laundry and dishwasher detergents—are loaded with chemicals that can pose a threat to human health, especially the health of children. Doesn't it make sense to get rid of these potential toxins as early as possible—ideally, before your child is even conceived?

In a 1996 survey, the EPA found that 74 percent of U.S. households were using one or more pesticides in the home. And conventional household cleaners—from chlorine bleach-based detergents to drain cleaners—have been linked to a staggering range of illnesses, especially childhood illnesses, from asthma to cancer.

Eliminating toxic household cleaners can greatly improve your home's indoor air quality, which has become a major health issue in recent years. Indoor air pollution—which can be two to five times worse than outdoor air pollution—has contributed to a rise in childhood respiratory disorders, including asthma and allergies. In fact, for the past seven years, the EPA has ranked indoor air pollution as one of the top five risks to human health. And according to the World Health Organization, approximately 30 percent of buildings have serious indoor-air quality issues.

The air in our homes might contain any number of toxins—dust mites; bacteria; particles from cooking, cleaning, smoking, and pet dander; pollutants brought in from outdoors like pollen, pesticides, and heavy metals—that can reduce our ability to perform mental tasks and even contribute to diseases as serious as cancer.

By greening your cleaning, you are also reducing your everyday exposure to these toxins, which have been linked to numerous childhood health problems, everything from ADHD and asthma to birth defects and reproductive problems. Waste no time in replacing your toxic products with environmentally friendly alternatives. These and other ingredients in conventional household ingredients might be doing real damage to your health:

Aerosol propellants, which can be found in conventional oven cleaners, carpet cleaners, furniture polishes and waxes, air fresheners, insecticides, upholstery cleaners, and spray starches, are eye, throat, and respiratory irritants that can aggravate asthma and cause other lung diseases. Exposure to aerosol propellants can also lead to eye injuries and chemical burns.

Alkylphenolic compounds, which are often a main ingredient in all-purpose cleaners and laundry detergents, are endocrine disruptors that have been shown to mimic the hormone estrogen and disrupt the body's hormone signals that regulate reproduction and development.

Ammonia, which can be found in conventional window cleaners, furniture polishes and waxes, and metal polishes and cleaners—is listed as a toxic chemical on the EPA's Community Right-to-Know list. It irritates the skin, eyes, and respiratory passages, causing all sorts of respiratory problems, including pulmonary edema. It is extremely toxic when inhaled in concentrated vapors and repeated exposure may lead to bronchitis and pneumonia. Ammonia can cause chemical burns, cataracts, and corneal damage and has been shown to produce skin cancer.

Chlorine bleach and chlorine byproducts form the basis of all sorts of conventional household cleaners: toilet-bowl cleaners, laundry detergents, dishwasher detergents, tub and tile cleaners—the list goes on and on. It's imperative that you stop exposing yourself to this dangerous respiratory irritant, which is one of the primary causes of household poisonings in the United States.

Formaldehyde, a carcinogen in humans, can be found in many conventional air fresheners, disinfectants, and spray starches. Exposure to formaldehyde can severely irritate or burn skin, eyes, nose, mouth, throat, and lungs, in addition to triggering skin allergies, asthma attacks, and even pulmonary edema. For more information on formaldehyde in other parts of the house, see page 40.

Perchlorethylene, or PERC, is a toxin found in spot removers, degreasers, and carpet cleaners. It's also the main chemical used in conventional dry-cleaning fluids. So if you're thinking about getting pregnant, I strongly suggest to find a nontoxic dry cleaner in your neighborhood, as PERC is a bioaccumulative toxin, meaning it can build up in our fat tissues. When inhaled by a pregnant woman, PERC can interfere with a developing fetus and also contaminate breast milk.

Petroleum distillates abound in just about every conventional consumer product on the market: lip gloss, perfume, hand dishwashing liquid, fertilizer, pesticides, plastics, paint thinners, solvents, artificial fragrances, furniture polishes, stain removers, and oven cleaners. If at all possible, try to phase these highly flammable bioaccumulative compounds out of your life, especially if you're thinking about having children. Exposure to petroleum distillates might pose risks to the liver, respiratory, cardiovascular, immune, endocrine, and gastrointestinal systems.

Benzene, a toxic emission of burning coal and oil, is a particularly dangerous petroleum derivative that has been implicated in incidences of childhood leukemia, the most common cancer in children. Tests on animals have shown that benzene can damage a developing fetus. The main sources of benzene exposure are tobacco smoke and vehicle exhaust, but toxic cleaning products might also put you at risk.

Toluene, another volatile organic compund, is a highly toxic petrochemical solvent. A carcinogen, neurotoxin, and eye and skin irritant, toluene is used in a staggering array of products used both to clean and to renovate the home: aerosol paints, floor polishes and other household cleaners, adhesives and sealants, paint and varnish removers, undercoats and primers, vinyl flooring, bathmats, waterproofing compounds, and industrial particleboard.

Phenol, often an ingredient in conventional laundry detergents, all-purpose cleaners, air fresheners, disinfectants and furniture polish, metal polishes and cleaners, fabric softeners and dryer sheets, is a known mutagen and suspected carcinogen. It can severely irritate or burn skin, eyes, nose, mouth, throat, and lungs. Phenol can also interfere with the ability of the blood to carry oxygen and cause bronchitis to develop. Higher exposures can cause a buildup of fluid in the lungs, which can lead to pulmonary edema. Internal consumption of large quantities can lead to circulatory collapse, convulsions, cold sweats, coma, and death.

Safe Alternatives

All over the country, safe, effective natural alternatives to conventional household cleaning products are becoming more available every day. As more and more of us clean up our lives, green alternatives will be even easier to find—and cheaper, too. Look out for products that disclose all ingredients (and tell you that they do).

You'll find that making the switch to nontoxic cleaners will save you a lot of money, since you'll no longer have to cram your cabinets with countless specialty products. Just a few basic cleaning products will suffice for most cleaning jobs.

1. **All-purpose cleaner** will clean floors, counters, kitchen surfaces, bathrooms, tubs, tiles, carpets, spills, and stains. Imus GTC (Greening the Cleaning) makes an extremely effective nontoxic all-purpose cleaner, which you can purchase at imusranchfoods.com and at thousand of stores nationwide. One hundred percent of the profits from sales of these products go to the Imus Ranch for kids with cancer. Seventh Generation (www.seventhgeneration .com), Sun & Earth (www.sunandearth.com), and other environmentally friendly companies also make nontoxic all-purpose cleaners.

2. **Window/glass cleaner** will clean glass, windows, and all stainless steel. GTC has an excellent nontoxic window cleaner.

3. **Automatic dishwashing detergent.** Seventh Generation (www.seventhgeneration.com) makes a good nontoxic automatic dishwashing detergent.

4. **Hand dishwashing liquid** will clean pots, pans, dishes, fine china, glasses, teapots, coffeepots, silver, and anything else you don't want to put in your dishwasher. GTC, Ecover (www.ecover.com), Earth Friendly (www.ecos.com) Sun and Earth, and Seventh Generation all sell safe dishwashing liquids.

5. **Laundry liquid.** GTC, Bi-O-Kleen (www.biokleenhome.com), Ecover, Earth Friendly, and Seventh Generation all offer great alternatives to conventional laundry liquids.

6. **Baking soda,** or sodium bicarbonate, is unbelievably useful in every room of your house. It can neutralize acid, scrub shiny materials without scratching, unclog and clean drains, extinguish grease fires, and remove certain stains. Baking soda can also be used to deodorize your refrigerator, carpets, and upholstery. It can clean and polish aluminum, chrome, jewelry, plastic, porcelain, silver, stainless steel, copper, and tin.

7. **White distilled vinegar** works much better than any toxic disinfectant you can buy. It contains about 5 percent acetic acid, which makes it great at removing stains. Vinegar can also dissolve mineral deposits, grease, remove traces of soap, remove mildew or wax buildup,

polish some metals, and deodorize almost every room of your house. You can use it to clean coffeepots, windows, brick, stone, carpets, toilet bowls—just about every surface in your house except marble, in fact. A tablespoon of white vinegar added to the rinse cycle also acts as a wonderful fabric softener. While it's normally diluted with water, in some cases it can be used straight. I recommend using organic vinegar, which is slightly pricier than the nonorganic kind but still a lot cheaper than most consumer cleaning products.

8. **Lemon juice** is a natural odor-eater that combines well with other ingredients. It can be used to clean glass and remove stains from aluminum, copper, clothing, and porcelain, and nothing works better on Formica surfaces. When exposed to sunlight, lemon juice is a mild lightener or bleach. Squeeze the juice from half a lemon into the wash cycle to get rid of odors on clothing.

9. **Table salt** is great at removing rust. With lemon juice, it can clean copper. When mixed with vinegar, salt polishes brass. Salt is also a key ingredient in an effective, all-natural scouring powder.

I also recommend keeping some hydrogen peroxide on hand, which in diluted form is great at removing stains from heavily soiled whites and other clothing and a number of surfaces. Essential oils (see page 160) are excellent disinfectants, and ketchup is useful for cleaning copper and brass.

And you only need a few basic supplies to maximize the efficacy of these environmentally friendly cleaners. First off, I recommend that you buy a microfiber mop, some washable microfiber cloths, and a microfiber duster. Microfiber is excellent at cleaning up messes, and because it's washable, you don't have to keep replacing your rags and mops every few months. If you do use paper towels, make sure that you buy only products that have been whitened without chlorine bleach, to guard against dioxin contamination. Green Forest (www.greenforest-products.com) and Seventh Generation (www.seventhgeneration.com) both make great eco-friendly—and price-competitive—toilet paper and paper towels.

You should also keep some scouring pads on hand (but not the ones that have been pretreated with toxic detergents), as well as natural cellulose sponges; a vacuum cleaner with a HEPA filter; gloves; a large scrub brush; old toothbrushes; and rags—yellowed old T-shirts or bar towels.

And that's it! You're done. Just find a few nontoxic cleaners you like and you'll be going a long way to protecting your family's health in the years to come. For a list of environmentally friendly household cleaning brands that I recommend, please turn to the Buying Green section on page 256.

However you choose to clean, make it a rule never to bring a product into your home without first thoroughly investigating its ingredients. Products containing chlorine bleach, ammonia, and petroleum distillates can all have serious health consequences for your family. Don't take the safety of anything for granted.

Green Building and Renovating

Ideally, if you're planning to renovate your home, you should finish construction before you even try to become pregnant. Fetuses and infants are extremely susceptible to toxins in the environment, which increase in concentration during household construction. Obviously, renovating in advance isn't always possible, but do keep these risks in mind as you plan your new home.

If it's not practical for you to renovate your home prior to pregnancy, you should try to stay away from the building as long as possible, preferably until construction is completed. If you cannot make arrangements to live elsewhere for the duration of construction, make sure that you have proper ventilation and that all materials and dust are cleaned before you reenter the building. Asbestos and lead dust from paint is particularly harmful during renovations. Other potential risks worth taking into account include:

PCBs, or polychlorinated biphenyls, are a chlorine-based chemical compound once used as coolants and lubricants in electrical equipment. Although PCBs have been banned since 1997, they still persist in our environment. Exposure to PCBs has been linked to reduced IQs in children, deficits in intellectual ability, and poor short-term memory and attention span. These compounds can be extremely toxic to the immune system. PCBs also disrupt thyroid hormone homeostasis, which is a crucial part of fetal development. The U.S. Department of Health and Human Services, EPA, and International Agency for Research on Cancer have all concluded that PCBs probably cause cancer. So if you have fluorescent lighting fixtures that are more than thirty years old, consider replacing them: They may be leaking PCBs into the air.

And be warned that another major source of PCB contamination is dietary. Non-organic fish, meat, and dairy products can all contain trace amounts of PCBs. According to the Agency for Toxic Substances and Disease Registry, women who ate large quantities of PCB-contaminated fish were more likely to have babies with reduced birth weights, behavioral problems, or impaired immune systems. A recent study of 212 fifth graders in Michigan suggests that prenatal exposure to even very low levels of PCBs can lower children's IQs.

Styrene, a petroleum distillate also known as vinyl benzene, has been classified by the EPA and Occupational Safety and Health Administration (OSHA) as a possible human carcinogen. Styrene primarily affects the central nervous system. Exposure might cause headaches, dizziness, confusion, and drowsiness, among other symptoms. A major component of indoor air pollution, styrene is found in many consumer products, especially those associated with home renovation: plastics, rubbers, resins, insulation, fiberglass, pipes, containers, wainscoting, and carpet backing. If you're thinking about remodeling your home, ask about the styrene content of the building materials you're considering using. A number of the most common—caulking compounds and sealants, vinyl flooring, and various paint-related products—might be worth avoiding.

Volatile organic compounds (VOC) are substances that contain carbon and different proportions of other elements such as hydrogen, oxygen, fluorine, bromine, sulfur, or nitrogen. Because VOCs become gases at room temperature, they're easily absorbed into our bodies. Perhaps the most famous example of a VOC, formaldehyde, has been banned in urea foam insulation, but formaldehyde is still used in many other consumer products, including paint-related products, household cleaners, vinyl flooring, adhesives, sealants, wall coverings, particleboard, and other renovation materials.

Greener Building Materials

Every month, it seems, another environmentally friendly alternative to traditional building materials comes onto the market. Do a little research to discover the ever-increasing pool of options now available to you.

Paint. There's nothing like paint to spruce up your home. But be aware that low-level exposure to many ingredients in traditional paint formulas can irritate or burn the eyes, nose, throat, and skin, as well as cause headaches, dizziness, or nausea. Luckily, you can easily reduce your exposure to the toxins found in ordinary paints. Companies are now offering low volatile organic compound (VOC) or odor-free paint, and some make paints that are completely free of VOCs. Look into these eco-friendly paint options:

Eco Spec by Benjamin Moore (www.benjaminmoore.com)

Safecoat by American Formulating and Manufacturing (www.afmsafecoat.com)

Ecological Paint by Innovative Formulations (www .innovativeformulations.com)

Benajmin Moore and AFM in particular have these healthier paints in a huge range of colors—a must-have for babies' rooms.

Flooring. First, avoid wall-to-wall carpeting if at all possible. It's a major contributor to indoor air pollution. If you love the feel of fabric under your feet, opt for easily washable area rugs instead. Vinyl—a chlorine byproduct made with petroleum distillates—is another potentially dangerous flooring material. Many other conventional types of flooring might contain products made from nonbiodegradable, nonrecyclable, and nonrenewable petroleum resources.

The good news is, in recent years, the flooring industry has introduced some more environmentally friendly alternatives. Bamboo, cork, natural fiber carpets, carpets made from partially or fully recyclable materials, reclaimed or rediscovered wood, and natural linoleum are among the many flooring materials now available to you. Refer to page 257 of the resources section at the end of the book for an extensive list of safe, attractive flooring options.

Lighting. Practical, energy-efficient alternatives to standard light bulbs, called compact fluorescent lamps (CFLs), are now widely available in a variety of sizes and shapes. Many CFLs produce light that has a warm appearance, similar to that given off by an incandescent bulb. Although larger than ordinary light bulbs, CFLs are getting smaller and will fit in many light fixtures. Newer models contain electronic circuitry that make them lighter and more compact, without the hum and flicker of ordinary fluorescent lights.

CFLs use one-quarter to one-third as much electricity as

incandescent bulbs and last up to ten times longer. They're also recyclable. In fact, because they contain mercury, CFLs shouldn't be thrown out in the trash If widely used, their environmental benefits would be enormous. Where electricity is produced from coal—and most is—each CFL will cut carbon dioxide emissions by about 1,300 pounds over its lifetime. For information of CFLs, visit Panasonic's Web site (www.panasonic.com/consumer_electronics/bp_lighting/ default.asp). GE (www.GElighting.com) also has answers to frequently asked questions about CFLs.

CFLs work best in light fixtures you tend to keep on for at least 15 minutes, and, of course, be sure to turn off standard light bulbs when lights aren't necessary. Your electricity bill will thank you!

Insulation. Traditional types of insulation can be irritating to the skin, nose, throat, and lungs. Conventional fiberglass insulation might contain formaldehyde, a known carcinogen. Natural insulation products such as cotton, cellulose, and straw bales are filling a growing niche in the insulation market. Consumers need to consider a full range of aspects concerning insulation, including energy efficiency, the environmental impact of raw material acquisition, product performance, flammability, and recycled content. At the Women's and Children's Pavilion at Hackensack, we insulated the walls with 117,000 pairs of preconsumer recycled denim jeans. For information on safer insulation, contact Bonded Logic (www.bondedlogic.com).

Rooftops and Ceilings. In the sweltering summer months, the temperature of conventional flat rooftops can rise up to 140 degrees Fahrenheit. This extreme heat creates updrafts that circulate tiny lung-clogging particles and also increases consumer electricity use. Green rooftops, by contrast, never get any hotter than 77 degrees. They also provide numerous environmental benefits. They filter air pollutants and retain as much as 50 to 70 percent of the storm water that they capture, which reduces both storm-water contamination and the risk of flooding. For more information on these innovative roofing materials, refer to the Institute for Research in Construction (http://irc.nrc-cnrc.gc.ca) and GreenGrid (www.greengridroofs.com).

Conventional ceiling materials can also be problematic since so many are manufactured using the carcinogen formaldehyde. Learn more about a new generation of ceiling materials that are being made with safe recycled materials at Armstrong (www.armstrong.com).

Greening Your Baby's Nursery

As I've already mentioned, you should try to do as many home renovations as possible prior to pregnancy. But I know how things work: As soon as you get pregnant, your nesting instinct will kick in. You'll want to transform your home to make space for the newest member of your family. Just be sure to examine every last detail of whatever room you've designated as your future child's nursery and work to minimize any potential health risks well ahead of time. Your goal in designing the nursery should be to reduce, to the greatest extent possible, your child's exposure to potentially harmful toxins.

- Peeling or chipped paint and wallpaper pose risks for young children, who might come into contact with toxins by licking the paint or sealant. Paint the room well in advance of the baby's arrival, preferably with one of the no-VOC or low-VOC paints mentioned earlier. (And if you're pregnant, obviously do not do the painting yourself!) Make sure the room is properly ventilated while it's being painted.

- Wall-to-wall carpeting might contribute to indoor air pollution. Even carpets made from nontoxic natural fibers have a tendency to retain dampness and absorb airborne toxins, which might irritate your baby's developing respiratory system.

- Minimize dampness and mold, both of which can encourage allergies and irritate your child's respiratory system.

- Avoid situating your nursery in a room with no windows or windows that won't open. Ventilation is crucial to the indoor air quality of a room, so make sure the windows are screened but still easy to open. The more outdoor air you can get circulating in there, the better.

- Like carpeting, heavy curtains and thickly upholstered furniture also have a tendency to absorb airborne toxins and breed allergies. Choose untreated wood furniture and wooden shutters instead.

- Make sure that the smoke detector near your child's nursery works.

Once you've taken care of these basics, you can get on to the business of designing the perfect nursery. Your baby's room should be first and foremost a place of refuge and safety, where he is protected, to the best of your powers, from the toxins so pervasive in our environment. If you follow these simple, common-sense guidelines, you can make that refuge a reality:

- Never, ever let anyone smoke in this space. I'm constantly shocked by how many expectant parents allow tobacco smoke in their children's environments. Cigarettes contain many chemicals that are known human carcinogens. When children are involuntarily exposed to these toxins, their respiratory systems suffer. Children living with a smoker were 27 percent more likely to miss school due to respiratory illness than kids in nonsmoking homes. And children exposed to two or more smokers were 75 percent more likely than children from nonsmoking homes to call in sick. In addition, asthma is more prevalent in children who reside with a smoker. So just say no. The air in your child's living space should be clean and uncontaminated.

- Position your child's room as far as possible from major appliances and other electronic equipment. The radiation from electromagnetic fields given off by household appliances has been linked to leukemia in young children. Keep all but the absolutely necessary electronics out of the nursery.

- Call an integrated pest management (IPM) specialist to ensure that your nursery is free of roaches and other pests that can trigger asthma and other childhood illnesses.

Crib Shopping: The BFR Problem

A crib is one of the first major purchases most of us make for our child—make sure you choose yours wisely. I recommend a crib constructed out of untreated wood, or wood with a natural finish. I would avoid bedding that has been treated with brominated flame retardants (BFRs), which are present in an alarmingly wide range of consumer products: TVs, computers, mattresses, carpets, kitchen appliances, paints, sheets, baby mattresses, and pajamas.

BFRs are added to prevent fires and reduce property damage, but scientific studies have raised concerns that they might also be contaminating wildlife and people on a large scale. Dr. Kenneth Bock considers flame retardants "a double-edged sword. You don't want something to catch on fire and have your kid burn," he said. "Obviously, that would be a tragedy. On the other hand, all these polybrominated flame retardants are really problematic. I'm concerned that these halogenated organic substances may be some of the things that are contributing to a lot of thyroid disorders in kids and adults these days."

Scientists are only just beginning to study the health effects of these persistent bioaccumulative pollutants, which are being manufactured in more astronomical quantities every year. Most people who've had their "body burden" tested for chemical exposures have had "huge levels of flame retardants," said Frances Beinecke. "And it's not from their own pajamas; it's from flame retardants that are used widely, whether in your car or the airplane you're travelling in. Obviously, you don't want to be on an airplane that hasn't been treated with flame retardants, should there be a fire. On the other hand, maybe there's a better product that serves the same purpose, without the same potential health impacts. And I think that's the direction that we have to be going in: pushing for alternatives in the marketplace that provide the same service but don't have the same chemical and health properties."

And the marketplace might in fact be moving in this direction. In response to growing health concerns, several major companies, like Dell, have committed to eliminating flame retardants from their products over the next few years. Until we understand more about these extremely high volume chemicals, we need to reduce our children's exposure to them whenever possible. While impossible to avoid altogether, flame retardants do not belong in the enclosed space where newborns spend the majority of their nights and days.

Safer Cribs and Bedding. You should definitely invest in an organic nontoxic crib, mattress, and sheets. For the best prices on healthy cribs, crib mattresses, bumpers, and other crib accessories, go to Organic Baby Mattress (www .organicbabymattress.com). If I were having another baby, I would order from here. These Amish-made cribs, hand-crafted in Ohio, are absolutely beautiful, entirely affordable, and completely nontoxic. Free of oils and chemicals, Organic Baby Mattress's whole line is compliant with the Consumer Product Safety Commission's fire codes. I especially love their Moses baskets, which is where Wyatt slept when he wasn't in his crib.

Other Furniture Retailers. A Natural Home (www .anaturalhome.com) has a great selection of natural kids' and baby furniture, including cribs, toddler beds, mommy rockers, changing tables, wooden play furniture, and natural wooden toys.

EcoBedroom (www.ecobedroom.com) makes wonderful wool puddle pads, which I used all the time with Wyatt. You place them in the crib, directly under your baby, and whenever your child wets his diaper, the wool puddle pad— and *not* the mattress or fitted sheet—absorbs the urine. I recommend buying several of these pads, which are much, much safer than a toxic plastic mattress cover. The wool pads are very easy to hand wash with a nontoxic laundry liquid. EcoBedroom also carries a varied selection of healthy baby bedding, mattresses, pillows, and furniture. EcoChoices (www.ecochoices.com), which is part of the same company, has a beautiful selection of baby blankets made from organic wool, cotton, and bamboo.

Greening Your Kitchen

In my family, we all love spending time in the kitchen. Cooking, eating, or just hanging out—we all just somehow gravitate to the kitchen. A green kitchen is an even more enjoyable place to spend time. You don't have to hire a contractor or spend a lot of money to transform your kitchen into a greener, healthier space. It's easy to enjoy the benefits of a green kitchen:

Maximize sunlight and ventilation. Nothing's more welcoming than a kitchen with a lot of big windows that let the sunlight and fresh air stream in. Natural sunlight can also reduce stress and improve your overall state of health. And as always, work to improve your indoor air quality by keeping the outdoor air circulating through your house.

Filter your water. We're exposed to tap water through so many different channels: juices and hot beverages, vegetables, the bath or shower, in the swimming pool, or even in the water you use to prepare food. Make sure that all of these sources are safe in your home—you might be in for an unpleasant surprise.

The Natural Resources Defense Council (NRDC) has found that millions of Americans drink tap water that may be contaminated with multiple biologically disruptive agents and toxic or cancerous chemicals such as lead, arsenic, pesticides, volatile organic compounds, radioactive materials, and agricultural herbicides. These toxins enter the groundwater via industrial processes and discharges from manufacturing facilities. Some scientists estimate that approximately 560,000 people each year become sick from contaminated drinking water, and kids drink more water per pound of body weight than adults, so they're at an even higher risk. Make filtering your water a priority.

If you have the money, I recommend installing an under-the-counter reverse osmosis system, which eliminates not only the chlorine but also the other toxins present in the water system. For the less expensive option, the Brita and Pūr filters—available at grocery stores nationwide—work pretty well, but you must change the filters regularly; otherwise, you defeat the whole purpose of having a filter. The Gaiam catalog (www.gaiam.com) has some devices for filtering water in the shower and bath.

And if you have kids already, know that fluoride could contribute to health problems that researchers are only just beginning to understand. While it does reduce cavities, fluoride might also promote much more serious health problems, including a rare bone cancer in boys. So get an inexpensive filter for your drinking water, as well as the water you use for bathing and cooking.

As much as possible, try to cut back on your bottled-water habit. Manufacturing these bottles consumes tremendous quantities of petroleum, and more than three-quarters of the 70 million bottles of water we purchase *every day* in this country go straight to the landfill, where they generate dangerous fumes. Filtering your own water at home is much better for the environment. If you're on the go and need to grab a bottle, try to buy one made out of #2 plastic, which is safer and more easily recyclable than other types. (You can find the number on the bottom of most containers.)

For detailed information on the best water filter options for your house, refer to the resources section.

Choose small, energy-efficient appliances. Purchase appliances with the Energy Star label. Energy-efficient home appliances use less water and electricity and they also cost a lot less to operate. You'll see a big difference in your electricity bill after you make the switch to Energy Star.

Opt for easy-to-clean surfaces. Grout can be a hassle. Low-maintenance counters and floors will save you a lot of headaches—and dollars—over the years.

Get rid of nonstick pots and pans. When overheated, the perfluorochemicals (PFCs) in Teflon and other nonstick substances can pollute our ecosystem and may threaten our health. Cook in cast iron or stainless steel instead.

Avoid plastic wraps and aluminum foil. Plastic and aluminum might leach toxins into the food you eat. To protect yourself, use waxed paper for covering food in the oven and refrigerator. And instead of plastic sandwich bags, we use brown wax paper baggies made by Natural Value (which you can purchase at www.amazon.com or www .shopnatural.com). I send Wyatt off to school with them every day.

Prepare organic whole foods for your family! In the chapters to come, and in the resources section at the end of this book, I offer lots of suggestions for healthy, nourishing foods that you can prepare in your kitchen in just a few minutes. Try out these ideas to improve the overall quality not just of your kitchen, but of your life.

I cannot emphasize enough the importance of having a welcoming, clean space for family meals. By taking charge of our children's relationship with food, we can revolutionize their whole future.

Chapter 4

Eating Right for Two

Nothing's more important than eating a nutritious, well-balanced diet before, during, and after your pregnancy. The foods you eat can be a powerful source of good or bad, of nourishment or deprivation. An unhealthy diet, especially in the first months of pregnancy, has been linked to reduced birth weight and head circumference, reduced intelligence, and increased risk of high blood pressure and stroke later in life.

As Joel Fuhrman told me, "A woman's diet prior to and during pregnancy is a critical part of childhood health problems, like autism and allergies and asthma and all sorts of brain and developmental disorders like ADHD. It's also what the kids eat when they're young, but it's also what happens to the developing egg and what happens in the womb. And I blame the American diet."

Never forget that when you're pregnant, you're really eating for two—your baby is actually using more than half of all the nutrients you're consuming. It's important that you take all the steps necessary to ensure that your baby is getting all the nutrients he needs to flourish. Your core diet should consist of a variety of nourishing whole foods, with a focus on the following categories:

- Unrefined complex carbohydrates. Buy more organic whole foods and whole grains: brown rice, millet, kamut, barley, quinoa, whole wheat, soba (buckwheat), and spelt.

- Organic fresh fruits, vegetables, and other plant-based foods naturally rich in nutrients. You should buy produce in season to reduce your risk of exposure to chemically treated produce.

- Calcium-rich foods (leafy green vegetables, oranges, bread).

- Fatty acids are essential for healthy membranes, hormones, and nerves. Load up on walnuts, pumpkin seeds, soybeans, linseed oil, rapeseed oil, and flax oil.

- Olive oil, sunflower seeds, almonds, corn, sesame seeds, safflower oil, and extra virgin olive oil are a source for linoleic acid.

- Garlic can lower blood pressure enough to reduce the risk of a stroke, coronary disease, and blood clots.

And just as you should go out of your way to load up on these healthy foods, you should be just as vigilant about avoiding certain foods, especially these:

- Fish, especially larger types that may contain high levels of mercury (see page 59).

- Alcohol (see page 62)

- Table salt and excessively salty foods

- Highly processed foods, food additives, and foods high in trans fats and chemicals.

- Meat. Meat-based diets have been linked to heart disease, colon cancer, and bladder and rectal cancers. In fact, women who eat red meat once a day have a 250 percent increased chance of getting colon cancer compared with women who eat it less than once a month.

- Estrogen mimics. Estrogen mimics are chemicals that our bodies perceive to be estrogen, a naturally occurring hormone that governs the development of female characteristics. Estrogen mimics pose a threat to human health because our bodies perceive them to be estrogen, which may disrupt our endocrine system. Estrogenic toxins enter our bodies through various paths, including through the foods we eat, particularly meat, poultry, and nonorganic high-fat dairy products.

- Corn. Corn is sneaked into a wide variety of processed foods in this country, so always read the labels. I would avoid any product that contains genetically modified (GMO) corn, because there are still questions regarding the long-term health effects of genetically altered foods on the human body have not been thoroughly tested.

- Sugar. Sugars are also sneaked into tons of different foods, especially foods marketed to kids. Again, study the labels carefully before buying. Avoid all artificial sweeteners and instead satisfy your sweet tooth with evaporated cane juice, stevia, agave nectar, honey, blackstrap molasses, maple syrup (grade B only; grade A might contain formaldehyde), sucanat, date sugar, and fruit juice concentrates. For more information on different types of sugar, I highly recommend Marion Nestle's book *What to Eat*.

In addition to following these essential dietary protocols, you should also take a prenatal vitamin to guard against certain birth defects. As early as possible, you should consult your health-care provider about which vitamins to take before and during pregnancy. Since folic acid helps prevent neural-tube defects and protects against preeclampsia, it's become standard practice for U.S. women of childbearing age to take a folate supplement.

Health-food stores carry a number of good prenatal vitamins, but you should always check with a professional before making your selection. It's crucial to get the dosage right. (Too much vitamin A, for example, can damage a developing fetus.) In this, as in so many other aspects of pregnancy, a good doctor will guide your decisions.

But be careful not to rely *too* much on vitamins. Instead, focus on getting as many of these nutrients as possible from the foods you eat. Folic acid, for example, can be found in kale, spinach, and other leafy greens. Broccoli, Brussels sprouts, cauliflower, green beans, cooked black-eyed peas, and baked beans also have a high folate content. Because the body can't store much folic acid, you must constantly replenish your supplies, so make these vegetables a staple of your prenatal diet. The prenatal vitamin is no substitute for good nutrition.

Joel Fuhrman cautions against relying too much on vitamins, especially during pregnancy. "We've turned everything into a pill," he said. The problem with giving women a vitamin to prevent birth defects, he said, is that some of them take this as a "permission slip" to ignore their diet, when "obviously any diet that's naturally rich in vegetables is very high in folate." Expectant mothers who take a folate vitamin and disregard other aspects of their diet usually end up deficient in "all sorts of phytonutrients and antioxidants." So remember, pregnancy vitamins should be a *supplement* to a healthy diet, not a substitute.

The ABCs of Organic Eating

Switching to organic food and beverages is an important step in detoxifying your body. "Eating organic food will reduce your exposure" to man-made chemicals, Dr. Kenneth Bock says. "And I know it's more expensive. But if you can go organic, you'll be eliminating things like arsenic and pesticides" and decreasing the overall level of toxins in your body.

For the longest-lasting results, make the switch to an organic diet gradually, one or two items at a time. Start with one of your favorite food items—apples, say. The next time you go to the grocery store, buy organic apples instead of your usual brand. Once you've become accustomed to these new apples, move on to another popular item.

Bit by bit, as you go along, continue to educate yourself about the benefits of eating organic. If the organic-foods aisle of your local supermarket leaves your head spinning, don't worry—you're not alone. Once you learn a few basics about organic food, you'll be able to shop for healthful foods for your family with no headache at all.

First, what does "organic" actually mean? Well, according to the consumer brochure of the USDA's National Organic Program, "organic meat, poultry, eggs, and dairy products come from animals that are given no antibiotics or growth hormones." Organic fruits and vegetables are grown and processed without the use of synthetic fertilizers or pesticides, many of which are known carcinogens and neurotoxins that have been linked to everything from cancer to learning impairments.

You should also bear in mind that the terms "organic" and "natural" are by no means interchangeable; don't be fooled by misleading labels. "Natural" can mean any number of things, while "organic" has a very specific, controlled definition. For a food to receive the "organic" label, a government-approved certifier must inspect the land where that food is grown to ensure that these USDA standards are being followed. You can't trust that a food is organic unless you see this label.

Now that you know the definition of organic, I can guess what you're probably thinking: But what if organic food costs too much? Do I have to buy *only* organic products?

These are completely legitimate concerns. While the prices of many organic foods have gone down over the last few years, many organic items still cost significantly more than the conventional alternatives. And while ideally you'd eat only organic foods, depending on your budget, you're sometimes going to have to pick and choose.

To help you prioritize, the Environmental Working Group has come up with a list of the twelve most important fruits and vegetables to buy organic. These rankings take into account the high pesticide residue levels found on the conventional versions. The produce items with the highest levels of pesticides are:

1. Apples

2. Bell peppers

3. Celery

4. Cherries

5. Grapes (imported)

6. Nectarines

7. Peaches

8. Pears

9. Potatoes

10. Red raspberries

11. Spinach

12. Strawberries

You can find a printable wallet guide of this list at www.foodnews.org/walletguide.php. And while you're on the Environmental Working Group's Web site, you should spend some time exploring other topics as well. You can access a wealth of useful information on a wide range of environmental issues, from drinking-water standards to carcinogenic ingredients in cosmetics.

For nonproduce items, the rules are even simpler. If you eat meat, eggs, and dairy products—which I don't recommend—you should only buy organic versions of these items, to protect yourself from antibiotics, growth hormones, and other dangerous toxins that nonorganic animal products all too frequently contain. So if you still want to eat meat, make sure that it's organic, grass fed, and free range.

Fish During Pregnancy: The Mercury Problem

Fish, especially fish from contaminated waters, can contain high concentrations of mercury, a neurotoxin that has been linked to lower IQs and can also hamper your ability to detoxify. More than 10 percent of women of childbearing age have levels of mercury that exceed EPA guidelines. High prenatal exposures to mercury can cause mental retardation, seizures, cerebral palsy, and vision, hearing, and sensory problems.

In the United States, emissions from coal-burning power plants are the number-one source of mercury in the environment. The mercury that these plants spew into the air ends up in our waterways, where it converts to methyl mercury and accumulates in fish, some at greater concentrations than others. The fish with the highest levels of mercury include:

- ahi or bigeye tuna
- tilefish

- swordfish

- shark

- king mackerel

- marlin

- orange roughy

When we eat those and other fish, we're essentially absorbing this fatal neurotoxin and teratogen (or, a substance that interferes with fetal development) into our bodies. During pregnancy, mercury can pass through the placenta into the blood—and brain—of the fetus we're carrying. Breastfeeding mothers with elevated mercury levels might also pass the neurotoxin on to their children. These exposures, however small, can give rise to lifelong brain and central nervous system problems in the affected kids.

Some forty-four states have issued advisories about eating mercury-contaminated fish. Women of childbearing age and children under the age of six are the population's most vulnerable to mercury's toxic effects. In 2004, the EPA and FDA issued a special advisory for pregnant mothers and women of childbearing age about mercury levels in mackerel and tuna.

But these measures aren't strong enough. The president of the Natural Resources Defense Council, Frances Beinecke, ranked mercury as one of her top two public health priorities. "Mercury is out there in the environment," she said. "The EPA put out a mercury policy last year, which we all think is incredibly inadequate. It isn't controlling mercury coming from coal-fired power plants, which is one of the major sources. And we have to be aggressive in demanding that mercury be controlled, just as sulfur dioxide and nitrogen oxides are controlled.

What we have now is not adequate. [The EPA's policy] needs to become much tighter, in order to protect kids' health."

Consider this: In 2005, a Centers for Disease Control and Prevention (CDC) report indicated that one out of seventeen women of child-bearing age has elevated blood mercury levels. In New York City, where sushi restaurants seem to be on every street corner, these levels are even higher: A recent report published in *Environmental Health Perspectives* (www.ehponline.org) found that the average blood mercury level of New York City women between the ages of twenty and forty-nine is *three times higher* than women in the same age bracket nationally. Asians and higher-income New Yorkers, who tend to eat more fish, have higher mercury levels. We don't yet know the full impact these concentrations will have on these women's children, but it can't be positive.

The good news is, if you cut mercury-contaminated fish from your diet at least six months before pregnancy, the mercury level in your blood can actually drop. So if you eat fish with any frequency and you're thinking of getting pregnant, you should really consider the potential effects the fish might have on your future child.

The FDA has found at least traces of mercury in nearly all fish. Although they say that eating some fish is safe, I recommend you avoid all fish for the duration of your pregnancy—the risks of contaminating your child with mercury are just too great. But to me, it doesn't make sense to give up fish during pregnancy and then resume eating it afterward. I recommend avoiding fish altogether. Pregnant or not, why would you want to contaminate yourself with mercury or other highly toxic bioaccumulative substances found in fish, like dioxins and PCBs? I wouldn't ever eat fish, period—at least not until we've cleaned up the mercury in our environment.

For more information on fish and mercury, visit the Natural Resources Defense Council's Web site, www.nrdc.org. The NRDC has the answers to many frequently asked questions about fish during pregnancy, as well as a mercury calculator and a consumer guide to mercury in fish (www.nrdc.org/health/effects/mercury/guide.asp).

Spotlight On: Fetal Alcohol Spectrum Disorders

To put it bluntly: Drinking alcohol during pregnancy is toxic to your child's development. Alcohol is a teratogen that can interfere with the healthy physical and functional development of a fetus at any stage of pregnancy.

Fetal alcohol spectrum disorders (FASD) is the country's leading known preventable cause of mental retardation and birth defects. Still, in the U.S., approximately forty thousand infants are born with incurable FASD every year—and all because women continue to drink alcohol when pregnant.

For almost thirty years now, we've known that alcohol, which can cross from the mother's bloodstream into the placenta, can interfere with fetal development. So my question is, why are expectant moms still drinking? And why are some doctors ignoring three decades of scientific research and telling pregnant women that the occasional glass of wine or beer is OK? If we know for a fact that drinking in large quantities can harm our babies, we can infer that small quantities will probably have a similarly negative impact. Like so many other disorders afflicting our kids today, fetal alcohol syndrome and fetal alcohol spectrum disorders are environmentally caused, meaning they are not a result of genetics.

To reduce the prevalence of fetal alcohol spectrum disorders, the biggest medical organizations in this country—the American Medical Association, the American Academy of Pediatrics, and the American College of Obstetricians and Gynecologists—have come together in advising women not to drink during pregnancy. Because so much of the damage takes place during the first trimester, women shouldn't even drink if they're at risk of becoming pregnant or trying to become pregnant.

I spoke with Dr. Kenneth Warren of the National Institute on Alcohol Abuse and Alcoholism about fetal alcohol syndrome (FAS) and the broader fetal alcohol spectrum disorders (FASD), a group of birth defects that are associated with drinking alcohol during pregnancy. Our most recent statistics, from a study published by the Institute of Medicine in 1996, estimates that every year, about 0.5 to 2 out of every 1,000 babies born in this country have fetal alcohol syndrome. Children with fetal alcohol spectrum disorders are not included in this figure, but Dr. Warren estimated that "probably about three times as many individuals have the broader FASDs than have the full FAS." Add it all up, and we're talking about significant numbers of children born every year with a 100-percent preventable birth defect!

Dr. Warren told me that, as opposed to many birth defects, like Down syndrome, fetal alcohol syndrome and fetal alcohol spectrum disorders can be very difficult to detect at birth, except in the most severe cases. While there are several other factors associated with FAS— growth impairment, reduced head circumference, and central nervous system impairment—doctors initially diagnose the syndrome on the basis of a unique combination of facial features, all of which can be too subtle to detect in a newborn baby.

According to Dr. Warren, these characteristic facial features—a combination of small eye width, thin, non-distinct upper lip, or the underdevelopment or absence of the "cupid's bow" and an elongated, non-distinct philtrum area (or the region with two parallel ridges between the upper lip to the base of the nose)—will only develop if a fetus is exposed to alcohol relatively early in the pregnancy. But, he went on, "even if a woman doesn't drink during the period when the facial features are developing, there's still a risk that all of the brain deficits—the

cognitive functioning and learning deficits—are still going to be there."
These children—who have all the same impairments in brain functioning as an FAS child, but not the facial features or even the impaired
growth—fall into a category known as "fetal alcohol spectrum disorders," which is even harder to diagnose than fetal alcohol syndrome.

So what amount of alcohol puts a developing fetus at risk for developing FAS or FASDs? By definition, "high-risk drinking" applies to
women who, on a drinking day, consume more than four drinks, probably exceeding the level of intoxication, which we define legally now in
most states as 0.08 blood alcohol concentration. While we know that
"drinking the same amount of alcohol in a short period of time, say
two hours, is a far greater risk than spreading that consumption out
over a much longer period," we don't yet have enough information to
determine the precise course of time over which high-risk drinkers consumed alcohol.

"Clearly," Dr. Warren told me, "the likelihood of having a child
with FAS, or of having a child that has an adverse result from alcohol,
increases with dose, and it really is a function of what we call quantity, frequency, and timing. It's the amount you drink, how often, and
when. There are clearly certain periods when alcohol is more dangerous," he said, adding that doctors don't yet know when all of those
periods are.

And even if we don't have enough data to determine if the occasional drink will harm your developing fetus, common sense suggests
that any amount of alcohol can be damaging. Just as your fetus breathes
through you, it drinks through you as well. Because a fetus is so small
and metabolizes substances more slowly than you do, the alcohol will
have a disproportionate effect on its development.

The good news is, even if you're a heavy drinker before you get
pregnant, as long as you kick the habit before conceiving, your child is
out of danger. "If a woman stops drinking before she gets pregnant," Dr.

Warren told me, "then she will have a healthy baby. We have individuals who've given birth to kids with FAS, but when they stop drinking, they then have healthy children. So the risk is really associated with drinking during pregnancy."

So play it safe. The less alcohol you consume during your child-bearing years, the better off your children will be. Give up all alcohol if there's even a remote possibility that you're pregnant.

Chapter 5

Pregnancy and Birth

W hy does it seem so difficult to have a healthy pregnancy these days? I've no doubt that the pregnancy complications we're increasingly seeing—from miscarriages to premature births—are linked to our toxic environment and the hectic pace of our lives.

The Healthiest Pregnancy Possible?

According to "The Faroes Statement," a recent peer-reviewed paper on the human health effects of developmental exposures to chemicals in our environment, "The periods of embryonic, foetal and infant development are remarkably susceptible to environmental hazards. Toxic exposures to chemical pollutants during these windows of increased susceptibility can cause disease and disability in infants, children and across the entire span of human life."

As I pointed out earlier, researchers haven't yet quantified the precise role environmental pollutants play in the growing number of birth defects we're seeing in this country; a recent estimate put the figure anywhere between 3 and 25 percent. We do know that roughly 2 to 3 percent of babies born today have a major birth defect, and about 18 percent of newborns are diagnosed with some minor structural anomaly.

Because scientists have only recently begun studying the links between these health issues and the environment, they don't yet know at precisely what age the critical exposures occur. There are several complicating factors to take into account as well. A fetus might come into contact with a toxin in the womb, but the consequences of this exposure might take years to emerge.

Chemical exposures might also increase the likelihood of a child being born prematurely (before the thirty-seventh week of pregnancy). In recent years, premature deliveries have risen steadily in this country, by more than 31 percent between 1981 and 2003, according to the March of Dimes. These days, nearly one out of every eight U.S. babies is born prematurely.

Dr. Michael Giuliano, chief of neonatology at Hackensack University Medical Center, offered several reasons for this steady increase in premature deliveries in this country, including various technological innovations. "Artificial technologies have led to lots of multiple births," he said, "and the incidence of prematurity in multiple births is much, much higher. In our unit right now, I think we have three or four sets of twins, just to give you an idea of how often—it's twins or triplets that actually make up a lot of the population."

But according to Stanford University pediatrician Alan Greene, the higher concentrations of chemicals in fetuses' blood might also be behind this increase. "The tiniest amount of pesticide increased the risk of prematurity by 90 percent," he said in a story in the *Dayton Daily News*, citing a University of North Carolina study conducted in the late 1990s, which evaluated forty thousand blood samples from pregnancies in the 1960s. "They went on to estimate that 15 percent of infant deaths in the 60s could be attributed to pesticide exposure before birth."

While researchers still have a great deal to learn about the causes of preterm delivery, the medical establishment widely acknowledges that preemies face greater challenges than full-term babies, from lung problems to neurodevelopmental challenges. In recent years, some re-searchers (including those from the Environmental Working Group) have even begun to link the rise in premature births to the obesity epidemic.

A Shortage of Sons

An explosive study released last summer by the University of Pittsburgh showed that over the last thirty years, in both Japan and the United States, the number of boys born for every 100 girls has declined from 105.5 to 104.5. This decline is "statistically significant," said Devra Davis, who headed the six-year study, since in most large societies, boy infants tend to outnumber girls slightly, at a proportion of 105 males to 100 females. Over the last thirty years, 5,000 fewer boys have been born for every million births.

"While it's a small decline for a population of three million in the United States, a little less in Japan, it does mean that we are missing baby boys," Davis said. "And as a population-wide phenomenon, you have to ask, 'What could explain this?'"

Though their evidence is not yet conclusive, Davis and her team of researchers have drawn a link between the reduced sex ratio and industrial chemicals, especially certain plastics and metals that have been proven to damage male-producing sperm. Heavy metals including arsenic, cadmium, lead, and mercury have been shown to affect the ratio of male to female births, and endocrine disruptors, like dioxin and PCBs, can play a role in determining a child's sex.

Regions with higher concentrations of these "gender-bending pollutants" in the atmosphere tend to have experienced a sharper decline in male births, as well as a jump in miscarriages of male fetuses. "In Minamata, in Japan," Davis said, citing one example, "they have reported that the biggest reduction in sex ratio in a population had been found where there was the highest level of mercury" after an outbreak of mercury poisoning in the late 1950s.

The University of Pittsburgh study, which was published in *Environmental Health Perspectives*, also mention a small Indian reservation in Canada that's surrounded by pipelines, factories, and petrochemical plants. In a region so dominated by the petrochemical industry that locals refer to it as "Chemical Valley," the 850 members of the Aamjiwnaang First Nation Reserve—many of whom work in the nearby factories—have experienced an alarming drop in the ratio of male to female births in recent decades. For every boy born in this small community, two girls are born—and the gap keeps on widening. Around 1993, the percentage of boys dropped below 50 percent, and that figure is now approaching 30 percent.

In an area with exceptionally high levels of dioxin, PCBs, pesticides, and heavy metals—all of which might interfere with a population's sex ratio—Aamjiwnaang children are suffering a multitude of other health problems as well. One in four has behavioral or learning disabilities, and these children suffer from asthma at nearly three times the national rate. Four of ten women on the reserve have reported at least one miscarriage or stillbirth. Now, when you look at these out-of-control numbers, you can begin to get a sense of the widespread damage these toxins are causing.

Our infant mortality rate is another issue of growing concern. According to a recent study conducted by Save the Children, the United States has one of the highest infant mortality rates in the industrialized world, with five deaths per one thousand births. Though we have more neonatologists and neonatal intensive care units than Australia, Canada, and Britain, we also have a higher infant mortality rate. American babies are 3 *times* more likely to die in the first month of life as children born in Japan and 2.5 times more likely than babies in Finland, Iceland, or Norway.

While many experts again link the increase in artificial technologies and multiple births, many feel that stress, poor nutrition, and alcohol abuse might also contribute. Limited access to health care is another problem, as is our lack of emphasis on prenatal care. "There's no protection for pregnancy," Dr. Manny Alvarez said. "We still have fifty million Americans without insurance. Women with limited insurance or who, for one reason or another, have to fall into, let's say, a clinic service, have long-term waiting periods. Many of these women have to wait a good number of months to see a doctor," he said, even *after* they know they're pregnant.

The earlier you can seek prenatal care, preferably in the first trimester, the better pregnancy outcome you're likely to have. There are other easy, common-sense steps you can take to protect your future children from birth defects, prematurity, and various childhood diseases.

Some Simple Guidelines

If you've already given up smoking and drinking and made a commitment to cleaning up your diet, you're off to a great start. Here are some other simple rules to live by during your pregnancy:

Try to stay in shape while pregnant. A regimen of regular but gentle exercise can make a big difference, both in your comfort level during pregnancy and in the health of your child. In her excellent book *Super Baby,* Dr. Sarah Brewer suggests exercising at a rate of about 70 percent of what you were doing before pregnancy, and even less as you enter the third trimester.

Exercise maintains good circulation, which allows blood and nutrients to reach your baby more effectively, and can lower the risk of miscarriage. Mothers who have stayed in shape during pregnancy have reported an easier time during labor, too; a fit mother tends to have a shorter labor, with fewer complications. Regular exercise will help you recover quickly after childbirth, and it can also increase your stamina and energy when you most need it—after the baby arrives.

Be careful, though, to avoid any overly strenuous activity, especially as your pregnancy progresses. Don't overdo it. Consider a prenatal yoga class to help you stay fit and manage stress during pregnancy. You can look for a prenatal class in your area or try a video at home (www.gaiam.com has a good selection). I also recommend taking regular walks during pregnancy; it's a great low-impact way to get more oxygen to your baby. If you'd like more tips on staying fit throughout your pregnancy, check out *Fit Pregnancy* magazine. And, as always, be sure to consult with your doctor about what type of exercise is right for you. You want to avoid anything too high impact.

Minimize stress. Pregnancy can be an emotional roller coaster. You're tired all the time, your hormones are out of control, you have a million things to take care of before the baby arrives. "We live in a very stressful society," said Dr. Manny Alvarez. "It's been shown that stress—just as it's been linked to high blood pressure and obesity—has also been linked to premature deliveries, because the chemical manifestation of stress is that it activates certain hormones in the body."

The baby that you're carrying inside you responds to your emotional signals, so go easy on yourself and turn down the anxiety levels. Stress can have a toxic effect on mothers and babies alike. According to *Super Baby*, mothers who are excessively stressed or anxious during pregnancy run a higher risk of giving birth to babies with low birth weight, small head size, or impaired neurological development.

If you feel overstressed, you should consider seeing a psychiatrist or therapist. I also found visualization techniques helpful during my pregnancy; there are many books on guided imagery available, including *Staying Well with Guided Imagery* by Belleruth Naparstek. Meditation, again, is an incredibly helpful way to control your stress levels during pregnancy. *Calming Your Anxious Mind: How Mindfulness and Compassion Can Free You from Anxiety, Fear, and Panic* by Jeffrey Brantley is a wonderful resource for women committed to bringing down their anxiety levels during pregnancy. *Calm Birth: New Method for Conscious Childbirth* by Robert Bruce Newman is a good introduction to a meditation program employed by many hospitals and birthing centers. The Calm Birth method prepares women for childbirth through breathing techniques and various other calming practices. Getting massages, either from your partner or a professional, will also help counteract stress.

Relax, recline, rest! Again, rest whenever you can. Dr. Sarah Brewer recommends leaving work between the twenty-eighth and thirtieth weeks of pregnancy, but that's obviously not an option for a lot of expectant mothers. As Dr. Alvarez pointed out, "Women have this fear: 'Oh, my God, I'm going to lose my job. I can't tell my boss [I'm pregnant] yet.' Then they come to me and say, 'My boss wants to know when you're going to deliver me.'"

If you're still working well into your third trimester, try to sit down as often as you can. When you're at home, lie down at frequent intervals to increase the blood flow to your uterus. You'll probably feel tired a lot of the time, especially in the later months of your pregnancy. That's fine—it's perfectly normal. Get as much rest as you need. Nap whenever you get a chance. Believe me, you'll be glad of the rest after the baby comes.

And if you work in a high-risk setting—at a dry cleaner or a nail salon, for example—consider finding an alternate job for the duration of your pregnancy. Parents whose jobs expose them to high concentrations of toxic chemicals tend to have higher levels of miscarriages and birth defects.

Don't get dental sealants or silver amalgams (fillings) when pregnant. Dental sealants can contain bisphenol A, a suspected endocrine disruptor, while traditional silver-colored fillings can contain as much as 50 percent mercury. But I don't advise getting any preexisting fillings removed, since the drilling part of the removal process can vaporize the mercury and actually increase your exposure to it. If you can't avoid dental work during this time, you should seriously investigate less toxic filling materials, like porcelain and gold. Talk to your dentist about viable alternatives.

Make intelligent choices about personal-care products. When you're pregnant, you shouldn't use any personal-care product that might harm your fetus, and that includes cosmetics. Your moisturizer, makeup, and deodorant all might be exposing your child to harmful chemicals. Go to www.cosmeticdatabase.com for a list of safe, and not so safe, personal-care products and cosmetics. This constantly updated Web site, provided by the Environmental Working Group, evaluates thousands of personal-care products— from shampoos to makeup to moisturizer—and rates them according to toxicity. It also lists which popular products might be cotaminated with impurities.

Products that may be contaminated with impurities.
9,747 (76.8%) products may be contaminated with impurities.
Showing top 20 product categories, ranked by prevalence.

Category	Percent of Products
Varicose/Spider Vein Treatment	100.0 (9)
Hair Color and Bleaching	98.1 (156)
Bubble Bath	97.4 (74)
Shaving Cream	96.2 (51)
Shampoo	96.2 (607)
Baby Wipes	95.0 (19)
Depilatory	94.3 (50)
Baby Sunscreen	93.8 (15)
Baby Shampoo	92.6 (25)

Category	Percent of Products
Mascara	92.5 (196)
Body Wash/Cleanser	91.8 (515)
Liquid Hand Soap	91.0 (81)
Baby Lotion	90.9 (30)
Sunless Tanning	90.5 (95)
Hair Spray	90.1 (127)
Hand Sanitizer	90.0 (9)
After Sun Product	89.7 (26)
Anti-aging	89.1 (197)
Moisturer	88.4 (1047)
Sunscreen/Tanning Oil	87.4 (250)

The vast majority of the personal-care products we use every day are packed with dangerous chemicals—some contact lens solutions, soaps, and detergents can even contain mercury—so do a little research before buying your next shampoo or moisturizer. Make a habit of buying 100 percent natural unscented, dye-free products, preferably ones in recycled or recyclable packaging, and opt for soaps and beauty products that contain no synthetic chemicals or dyes. And when you're pregnant, simplify your beauty routine—your natural glow is the only foundation you need!

Consider a natural birthing class. Some childbirth classes are more "natural" than others. For expectant moms committed to a completely natural, drug-free birthing process, the Bradley Method (http://www.bradleybirth.com) is an excellent resource. The Bradley Method teaches expectant moms holistic nutrition, exercise, and meditation, all information that will come in handy throughout your pregnancy. The Calm Birth (www.calmbirth.org) method, which has practitioners all over the country, is another option for mothers interested in giving birth naturally. Birthing from Within (www.birthingfromwithin.com) is another method worth exploring.

You might also consider hiring a doula to help you during labor. For more information on doulas, see Dona International's Web site (www.dona.org).

If you've taken all of these steps in the early months of your pregnancy, you've gone a long way toward protecting the health of your child.

Choosing the Right Hospital

Take some time to consider where you're going to give birth. If you're not planning to do a home birth, you should choose a green hospital or birthing center, like the one my environmental center helped to build at the Hackensack University Medical Center. The Sarkis Gabrellian Women's and Children's Pavilion, which opened in early 2006 after five years of research and planning, represents my vision of a healing hospital environment. With its the recycled denim insulation, natural rubber floors, and low-VOC paints, adhesives, and sealants, this 300,000-square-foot facility has been widely recognized as a pioneering achievement in green building. We've filtered the water, used recycled construction materials, found alternatives to PVCs, and installed energy-efficient lighting. But more than that, we've tried to make every element of the pavilion as inviting as possible. We've put plasma televisions in every patient's room. The dining area looks more like a trendy Manhattan restaurant than a hospital cafeteria. We've chosen a welcoming palette of pastel paints for every floor.

Obviously, Hackensack is way ahead of the curve here, but if you live in a metropolitan area, you can probably find a birthing facility with some of the same elements: nontoxic, or low-toxic, building materials; organic layettes for the baby and organic bathrobes for the mom; a healthy menu; nontoxic cleaning supplies; and birthing rooms with midwives. Some of the chemicals used in hospitals can be toxic and may pose dangers to newborn babies. According to the American Academy of Pediatrics' Green Book, "Epidemics involving absorption of chemicals through the skin in newborns include hypothyroidism from iodine in Betadine scrub solutions, neurotoxicity from hexachlorophene, and hyperbilirubinemia from phenolic disinfectants used to clean hospital equipment."

If you're interested in learning more about your birthing options, do some online research. You can find information on freestanding birthing centers (for example, www.greenhousebirthcenter.com) as well as women's stories about their experiences at freestanding birthing centers (http://centralfloridagreenguide.com/?s=birthing+cottage+winter+park). Some hospitals have their own birthing centers, with a midwife and sometimes a doula to assist. To find a midwife in your area, you can start at the American College of Nurse-Midwives' homepage (www.midwife .org/find.cfm).

Whatever you do, think through this decision carefully. Do your utmost to give birth in a soothing, nurturing, healthy, and relaxing environment.

Chapter 6

Developing Your Baby's Palate

For all the cultural transformations we've undergone over the last half century, none has been so dramatic as the way we eat. The rise of fast-food chains has had a huge impact on our eating habits. Since we're often too busy to cook at home, we grab processed foods out of the freezer and pop them into the microwave. We've been conditioned to want our food cheap, quick, and filling—no matter if that food also happens to be packed with triglycerides and trans fatty acids and artificial chemicals.

For the sake of our children, we need to start rethinking this damaging relationship with food, if possible at the very beginning of their lives. Poor nutrition plays a *huge* role in the health issues that we're seeing in our kids—it's no coincidence that our children's health has deteriorated with our diets. Feeding our kids a nutritious, well-balanced diet could solve a lot of their health problems right off the bat.

Our appalling diet has contributed to an epidemic in childhood obesity. In the modern world, very few parents take the time to cook anymore. We're too busy, or we've simply gotten out of the habit. In many families, both parents work, coming home just in time to zap some frozen dinner in the microwave. It's considered a luxury to be able to prepare healthy, nutritious, whole-food meals for our families.

As a result, our kids' health is suffering. About one in six children between the ages of six and nineteen is considered overweight. Overweight children and teens may be at risk for cardiovascular disease, including high cholesterol, elevated insulin levels, and elevated blood pressure. Overweight children and teens are also at a much higher risk of coming down with various chronic diseases later in life, including hypertension, type 2 diabetes, and coronary heart disease.

"The metabolic groundwork for the degenerative diseases of adulthood are really laid down in childhood," Dr. Michael Rosenbaum, associate professor of clinical pediatrics and medicine at Columbia University's College of Physicians and Surgeons, told me. "The interactions between the environment and any inherited (genetic) risk of these degenerative diseases really begins at the moment of conception and continues through childhood. You can't dismiss prenatal care or the way in which your child eats or exercises as 'unimportant.' Good prenatal care avoids fetal overnutrition, both of which carry an increased risk of adult disease," he said. "Childhood feeding and exercise patterns, which are largely determined by parents and the examples they set, have potent effects on disease risk and on adult health-related behaviors."

The problem is fairly simple: Our kids don't know how to eat right. The reason they don't know how to eat right is also simple: Because we've never taught them. Often, we don't know how to eat right ourselves, but it's long past time that we learned.

Changing our kids' diets isn't very difficult—that's not the problem here. After all, kids eat what their parents give them to eat. Their tastes develop according to the foods we give them, and their eating habits tend to carry over into adulthood. More than that, diet plays a key role in the development of a healthy immune system and a healthy brain and central nervous system.

And bear in mind that it's not just what we're putting *in* our bodies, but what we're *not* putting in. Nutritional deficiencies can leave children vulnerable to a whole host of health problems. Dr. Joel Fuhrman put the issue bluntly when he said, "I believe that the biggest exposure our cells get to the environment is through food. It's normal for the body to be exposed to some degree of toxic and carcinogenic materials," he went on, "because a body that's well nourished has the ability to detoxify toxic compounds and move them out of the system." Malnourished bodies lack that ability, which is one reason we're seeing so many diseases in childhood.

"I think the most dangerous things to feed children," Dr. Fuhrman said, "are potato chips and French fries and donuts and trans-fat-containing sweets and sausages and luncheon meats, pickled, smoked, and barbecued meats. These things that we call 'kid-friendly foods' and put on the kids' menus are in fact the most dangerous foods we can feed children."

Dr. Fuhrman wasn't the only doctor I interviewed who commented on these disturbing trends in children's diets. "It's not as if we're finding a 'deficiency' as we'd normally define it, but kids are not eating fresh foods," Dr. Frederica Perera said. "Frozen processed food transported from other countries is simply not as healthy as the diet of previous generations."

Many children are overnourished and yet deficient in most essential vitamins and minerals. "They're deficient," said Dr. Kenneth Bock, "in multiple nutrients—zinc, selenium, magnesium, essential fatty acids, and so many of the fat-soluble vitamins, like the vitamin A."

"Rather paradoxically," Dr. Phil Landrigan said, "you have the problem of overnutrition, or terrible nutrition. All the fast foods that people eat—the fatty foods, the sodas that kids drink by the gallon—have caused the trebling in the frequency in childhood obesity in the last fifteen years and the epidemic of diabetes which followed." As for the long-term outcome of these health problems? According to Dr.

Landrigan, it couldn't be bleaker: "The current generation of children is probably going to be the first generation in the history of the United States, for as long as we've been keeping national records, who will have a shorter life expectancy than their parents."

There's no excuse for bad nutrition, not when you consider all the diseases it can cause. To reverse these alarming trends, we should be feeding our children nourishing, delicious whole foods, foods that strengthen their developing bodies. Our children's diets—and beyond that, their relationship with food and eating—is absolutely within our control. We should be feeding our children foods that can regulate their metabolism, blood sugar, and even mood swings, hyperactivity, and depression.

The hard part, it seems, is for parents to change their *own* relationship to food. According to Dr. Rosenbaum, "Numerous studies show that good or bad health and exercise behaviors learned in childhood are more likely to persist into adulthood. You can lay the behavioral groundwork for good health earlier—just as you can alter the early metabolic groundwork for disease. It's very hard to change someone's behavior as an adult.

"In all the work I've done in the schools," Dr. Rosenbaum continued, "the hardest thing is to get the parents to come in" and learn about a healthier lifestyle.

Trust me, I know how hard it can be to change old habits. We all have strong cultural, and emotional, attachments to the foods that we eat and love. But if your favorite foods happen to be unhealthy, you need to make an effort to phase them out of your diet. Just try to bear in mind what's at stake: our children's health and the future of our society. So first and foremost, you have to overhaul *your* diet. In order to teach your family how to eat better, you must learn to eat better yourself.

A well-balanced diet is the basic foundation of good health that you can give your children, and the best moment to develop their palates is at the very beginning of their lives. "Food is a powerfully addictive substance," Dr. Fuhrman said. "But once you start eliminating all the sugars and transfats and unhealthy additives, you'll find that you get *more*, not less, pleasure out of the foods you eat."

As a family, make an effort to rekindle this pleasure. Eating shouldn't be a rushed obligation, something to be gotten over with as quickly as possible. It should be, as Dr. Fuhrman said, a pleasure, a reliable source of enjoyment and family togetherness. However frenzied our schedules, we can still prepare simple, wholesome meals without wasting time or breaking the bank.

By rejecting our culture's pervasive McDonald's mentality, we can make a huge difference in our children's futures. So from the very beginning, keep your kids away from junk food. Give them healthy sandwiches with fruit instead of candy, and water instead of sodas. And you don't have to sacrifice comfort foods, either—you can make healthy antioxidant pizza. Slowly replace white rice with brown rice. And get your kids involved in the kitchen—show them how to chop up kale and crush garlic. Make mealtimes a pleasurable, relaxed experience for the whole family.

Nursing

Immediately after childbirth, you face your first big decision about that baby's diet: to breastfeed or not to breastfeed?

We all know about the immunological benefits of breastfeeding. Breastfeeding can protect newborns from ear infections and other allergies. But in recent years, a new side has emerged to the breastfeeding debate: What about all the toxins the average childbearing-age woman is carrying around inside her? Are they contaminating the baby through breast milk? In recent years, the Environmental Working Group's staggering findings have raised a number of doubts about the benefits of breastfeeding. Various toxins, like mercury, have been shown to pass into a mother's breast milk.

In light of these findings, people have begun to ask, Is it safe to expose newborn babies to so many toxins? Do the threats those exposures pose outweigh the benefits of breastfeeding according to AAP's *Pediatric Environmental Health* guidebook, the American Academy of Pediatrics, the World Health Organization, and the U.S. surgeon general "have considered the problem of environmental contaminants in human milk and continue to recommend breastfeeding."

Many integrative physicians, like Kenneth Bock, M.D., likewise recommend breastfeeding whenever possible. "But you have to recognize that breastfeeding is a double-edged sword," Dr. Bock said. "You've got the healthful aspects of breastfeeding, which I support, but you must recognize that even in breast milk, there will be toxins." He went on to discuss the psychological and emotional benefits of a mother breastfeeding her child.

"Maybe I'm old-fashioned," he said, "but I still think that there's a value to that. I think if we do the other steps first—if we do the preconceptual and really clean up and detoxify as much as possible before giving birth—if that became the norm, then breast milk would become less toxic."

Dr. Lawrence Rosen, a groundbreaking integrative pediatrician and the medical adviser to our environmental center, agrees with this advice. "Most of us in primary care still advocate breastfeeding as ideally preferable to formula feeding," he wrote to me. "But with the addition of common brand organic formulas with added essential fatty acids and, in some cases, probiotics, the boundaries are blurring. I know this is controversial, but these are real-life questions families are dealing with today." In conclusion, he wrote, "Perhaps the ideal situation is trying to ensure that breast milk is as nontoxic as can be."

Open the dialogue with your obstetrician; discuss whether the immunological benefits of breastfeeding still outweigh the potential risks these chemicals might pose. Look into these organic formulas, which might be a good option for you. Dr. Rosen recommends discussing these organic formulas with your doctor:

- Similac Organic (www.similacorganic.com), with cow's milk

- Earth's Best Organic Infant Formula (www.babyorganic .com)

- Nature's One Baby's Only Organic (www.naturesone .com), with cow's milk or soymilk

- Ultra Bright Beginnings Organic (www.brightbeginnings .com/products/organic-baby-formula.asp), with cow's milk

Because the lipids in formula are derived from coconuts and other vegetable sources, they don't contain the kind of scary chemicals—including DDE, PCBs, hexachlorobenzene, and various industrial pesticides—found in human breast milk. Even women who haven't been occupationally exposed to these chemicals might be contaminated, so be careful.

If you do choose to breastfeed your child, you should be all the more vigilant about detoxifying your body before getting pregnant. Exercise regularly, stay hydrated and consume only the purest, most nutritious foods. The nutritional content of your diet will make a big difference in the quality of the milk you're feeding your child.

And while breastfeeding, you also need to monitor chemical exposures from personal-care products as well. Wear only phthalate-, paraben-, and chemical-free makeup, and use only nontoxic lotions, deodorant, face cream, face cleanser, shampoos, and other products. You want to limit your contact with all potenital toxins while you're nursing,

so I'd also avoid synthetic perfumes or nail polish. And consider investing in organic nursing pads and organic bedding for yourself as well
as for your baby—again, all of these minor routes of exposure might
increase the level of contaminants in breast milk.

You should also talk to your doula, midwife, and doctor about
using Weleda baby care products on you and your baby while breastfeeding, particularly Weleda Nursing Tea. And if you have any questions or concerns about breastfeeding, contact La Leche League (www
.lalecheleague.org). Their resources include mother-to-mother forums,
podcasts, and online help forms. La Leche League's classic book *The
Womanly Art of Breastfeeding* is updated frequently.

Another useful book on breastfeeding, Sheila Kippley's *Breastfeeding and Natural Child Spacing: How Ecological Breastfeeding Spaces Babies,* might interest mothers who've adopted the "attachment parenting"
approach. And last but not least, in her wonderful memoir of motherhood, *Having Faith,* Sandra Steingraber explores both sides of this
complicated issue: whether it's safer in the long term to breastfeed or
formula-feed her newborn.

Better Bottles

The popularity of clear, hard-plastic baby bottles made from
polycarbonate has skyrocketed in the last decade. These bottles are
available in a range of trendy shapes and sizes that parents love. But
what many parents don't realize is that these bottles are made with the
chemical bisphenol A (BPA), which can leach into baby's drink.

Consumer Reports was one of the first U.S. publications to cover
this topic for general audiences in the late 1990s, but despite this and
other news stories in past years, clear baby bottles still dominate store
shelves.

In February 2005, the nonprofit group Environment California released data on tests conducted on polycarbonate baby bottles. Although industry representatives have continued to insist that these bottles are safe, these studies are clearly cause for caution. The results reinforce other data showing that new polycarbonate bottles leach small amounts of BPA, which in animal tests has been shown to cause "abnormalities in the mammary and prostate glands and the female eggs of laboratory animals" as well as accelerating puberty and adding to weight gain.

What's even scarier: Every year, we produce 6 billion pounds of BPA, which is also found in some hard plastic water coolers, water bottles, microwave-safe dishes, even inside the linings of tin cans. We're exposed to it around the clock. A recent CDC study found that 95 percent of the people it tested had been contaminated with this chemical compound.

As with so many toxins, exposure to BPA is most dangerous early in life. According to Dr. Frederick vom Saal of the University of Missouri-Columbia, fetuses and newborns exposed to BPA even at low doses have a higher likelihood of developing prostate and breast cancer later in life. So make an effort to reduce your child's contact with BPA by choosing healthier baby bottles. BPA-free bottles include Evenflo glass bottles, which are available at major retail stores and select supermarkets. When Wyatt was a baby, glass bottles were a lot harder to find than they are now. I ended up ordering two dozen from the only source that stocked them, and I never broke a single one. Glass bottles are much safer, and unlike plastic, they last a long time, so you end up saving money. When Wyatt had outgrown his bottles, I passed them along to my sister, who used them with both her daughters. All she had to replace was the silicone nipple.

If you still prefer plastic, Born Free (www.newbornfree.com) makes bisphenol A–free clear plastic bottles, which you can buy on their Web site or at select Whole Foods stores. These bottles might cost a little more than the traditional, BPA-containing bottles, but I think it's an expense most parents would consider legitimate.

Remember never to heat any food or drink in plastic, including plastic wraps. The safest way to heat items is on a ceramic or glass plate or container. A baby's bottle can be heated under warm running water or with a bottle warmer.

You should also avoid pacifiers with plastic nipples. Instead, look for silicone nipples, which are easy to find at most baby stores. Latex nipples are also an option, but only if your baby isn't allergic—in general, I think silicone is safest.

Organic Baby Food

Sales of organic baby food have soared over the last few years. Since 1995, when the Environmental Working Group reported finding sixteen different pesticides (including three carcinogens) in baby foods manufactured by eight different companies, more parents have started thinking twice about the kinds of prepared foods they bring home to their babies. The giant of baby-food makers, Gerber, has introduced a new organic line, and several smaller companies have started to gain prominence in the supermarket aisles.

Despite these encouraging changes, organic baby food does still cost about 25 percent more than nonorganic baby food. If you're concerned about this price difference, shop around for specials at your local health-food store. You could also consider buying in bulk. Several companies, like Earth's Best (www.earthsbest.com), offer discounts if you purchase baby food by the case. It's worth doing that extra bit of work to protect your kids from a major source of pesticide exposure. Other companies making great organic baby food include Plum Organics (www.plumorganics.com), Happybaby (www.happybabyfood.com), Homemade Baby (www.homemadebaby.com), and Sweetpea Baby Food (www.sweetpeababyfood.com).

You can do your own exploring in the baby-food aisle and the frozen-foods section of your local health-foods store—but remember, always read the labels and look for that all-important USDA organic seal. And do an online search for organic baby-food merchants in your area, since many local companies offer delivery services. Even better: learn how to make your own organic baby food.

> *I nursed my baby, Noah, for eleven months, then he weaned himself. I then started him on Rice Dream original. He has never had an ear infection, flu, or any other health problem. Noah has never had any medication to date. Teething was handled with Hyland's Teething Tablets or chamomile tea at night, not Tylenol! The only dairy he has ever had is organic yogurt, frozen yogurt, or kefir.*
>
> *Another lifesaver is making baby food. Our household has a veggie mix, which is a great way to add many fruits and vegetables into every meal. Actually making up different recipes for Noah sparked interest for my husband and me to try some ourselves. Now the entire family makes a conscious effort to have at least seven fruits/veggies a day.*
>
> *Noah never had cradle cap or eczema. I used bath products that were free of irritants like propylene glycol or sodium lauryl sulfates. Products like California Baby and Burt's Bees are great. I especially loved Burt's Baby Bee Diaper Ointment! Massages with pure jojoba oil are great, too! I consider all these things "no-brainers," but I guess not for a lot of mothers, because there are so many bad and toxic products on the market.*
>
> Julie S., Dallas, GA

Got Milk?

Earlier in the book, I discussed making informed choices about which organic products to buy. In an ideal world, you'll bring only organic foods into your home. In reality, this isn't always possible. Sometimes, you'll be forced to pick and choose, to prioritize. Once your child is no longer breastfeeding, you'll face one of these choices. Should you give your child dairy products or not?

I strongly recommend that you discuss with you physician the idea of raising your kids dairy free. Nonorganic milk might contain any number of toxins that can impair your child's development: estrogen mimics, hormones, steroids, antibiotics, and even dioxin. In 1988, the Food and Drug Administration found that 73 percent of milk samples from grocery stores in ten different cities contained pesticide residues.

While you may have been led to believe that milk is necessary for strong bones and teeth, it may not be good for you or your children. Still, if you do decide to give your child dairy products, I strongly recommend that you go organic.

Let's take a closer look at some of the potentially dangerous substances that might be present in nonorganic cow's milk:

- **Growth hormones.** Many dairies treat cows with manufactured hormones such as recombinant bovine somatotropin (rBST). "Beyond Pesticides," a 1996 study published in the *International Journal of Health Services,* reported that milk from cows injected with recombinant bovine growth hormone (rBGH), a synthetically produced hormone that makes cows produce more milk, contains increased levels of a growth factor that has been linked to breast and gastrointestinal cancers in humans. Recombinant bovine growth hormone may also increase levels of the bovine IGF-1 growth factor. An increase in IGF-1 may provoke cancer cells to increase more rapidly and contribute to lung, colon, prostate, and breast cancer. Although the FDA says that there is "no significant difference" in cows treated with artificial hormones, you can find many dairies that refuse to use rBGH; look for milk producers who disclose on their labels that they don't use artificial hormones.

- **Dioxin.** Dioxin is the most carcinogenic substance *ever* tested. In addition to cancer, dioxin exposure has been linked to birth defects, inability to maintain pregnancy, decreased fertility, reduced sperm counts, endometriosis, diabetes, learning disabilities, immune system suppression, lung problems, skin disorders, lowered testosterone levels, and many other problems. Dioxins accumulate in fat cells, and have been found in fat-containing milk.

Women who eat dairy animal products and dairy products in particular might be five times more likely to have twins (and the risk for pregnancy complications that come with multiple births) than vegan women, according to a May 2006 study in the *Journal of Reproductive Medicine*.

And in a study published in the July–August 2007 issue of *Harvard Magazine*, even cows that haven't been fed bovine growth hormones might produce milk that has adverse effects on human health, since the milk-producing cows are kept pregnant and lactating for three hundred days a year. The result: higher than normal estrogen levels in the milk we drink. While we don't yet know the full impact of these exposures, researchers have linked unnatural concentrations of estrogen and other hormones to a number of cancers, including breast, testicular, ovarian, and uterine. Ganmaa Davaasambuu, the Mongolian physician and re-searcher who published this report, found that rats fed low-fat milk were "more likely to develop tumors, and in greater numbers and of larger size, than rats fed water or artificial milk."

Alternatives to Milk Products

Luckily, there are lots of great alternatives to conventional milk products. Sample the following products and pick your favorite:

- Soymilk (my favorite is Edensoy)
- Rice milk
- Coconut milk
- Almond milk
- Tofu buttermilk

Rice and soymilks are the most popular and readily available of these "milks," and they come in a variety of flavors, as well as in both conventional and organic. As always, I recommend you go organic whenever you can.

For more information on the benefits of a dairy-free lifestyle, please visit www.notmilk.com. VegWeb (www.vegweb.com) is another useful Web site, providing information on alternatives to other popular dairy products, like cheese and sour cream. VegWeb also has great vegan and vegetarian recipes.

Carrageenan

Carrageenan is used as an emulsifier, or thickener, in many different foods: baked goods, frostings, dairy products, processed cheeses, chocolate milk, jams and jellies, pie fillings, relishes, barbecue sauces, yogurt, pimento olive stuffing, and some soy milks, including the best-selling soymilk in America, Silk Soymilk. A 2001 study published in *Environmental Health Perspectives* showed that *degraded* forms of carrageenan can cause serious gastrointestinal problems, including ulcerations and gastrointestinal cancers. Even the undegraded forms found in most food products aren't altogether safe, as stomach acids and digestive enzymes can convert it into the more dangerous, degraded type. So if you or your child is allergic to dairy or soy, you might actually be allergic to the carrageenan.

So switch to a soymilk that doesn't use the additive, like Edensoy (www.edenfoods.com), or 8th Continent (www .8thcontinent.com), which uses cellulose gel and soy lecithin.

A Word on Microwaves

The demands of modern life never let up. We all work and drive carpool and juggle multiple competing demands. We come home exhausted and just want to put something hot in front of our kids every night, and here's where our trusty microwave comes in. We can toss just about any food in there and within five minutes be sitting down to eat.

I'm the first to acknowledge that microwaves are affordable and ultraconvenient. They save tons of time, but at what cost? Processed foods made for the microwave are junky, filled with trans fats and so-dium and hydrogenated oils, all of which are depriving our children of the nutrients they need to perform well in school.

Microwaves support the unhealthy lifestyle that is making our kids so sick. Take that little bit of extra time every day; I promise it will pay off in the long run. Your whole family will benefit if you make more of an attempt to nurture your bodies and spirits. Even if you're having frozen pizza for dinner, why not heat it for twenty minutes in the oven instead of zapping it for ninety seconds in the microwave? It takes longer, true, but the final product is much more nourishing and tasty—not soggy and rubbery like food that has been nuked to death in the microwave.

Microwaves are a perfect example of Americans' obsession with convenience above all else—our insistence on taking shortcuts, even at our own peril. We want everything both ways, all the time. We love food, but we're too lazy to prepare it or even to wait for it to heat up. We want our dinner right in front of us ASAP, in the snap of a finger.

We can't keep cutting all of these corners and expect to get away with it indefinitely. Our lazy habits are already beginning to catch up with us, as evidenced by the state of our children's health.

One easy step toward a healthier life is to get past your microwave dependence. If for some reason you don't already own a microwave, resolve never to buy one. Once you have a microwave, you'll find it very difficult not to use it constantly.

If after reading this you want to dispose of your microwave, do so responsibly. Microwaves are filled with PVCs and heavy metals and shouldn't just be tossed into the nearest landfill. Instead, take your microwave to the waste transfer station nearest your home. The EPA provides complete listings of regional waste transfer stations on its Web site (www.epa.gov/epaoswer).

If, on the other hand, you have no intention of ever getting rid of your microwave, at least take these simple precautions to minimize the health risks these machines pose:

- Your microwave should be positioned at the maximum possible height in your kitchen, at least at eye level. You absolutely don't want your reproductive organs soaking up any microwave radiation that may escape if your micro-wave has any leaks.

- Never microwave baby bottles.

- Never heat up food in plastic containers.

- Never cover food placed in the microwave, particularly not in plastic wrap.

Turn to the resources section at the end of the book for quick, easy snacks that don't require a microwave.

Blue Moon Treats

If you let your child stare at the computer or television screen all day, play on a Game Boy around the clock, live off chips and cookies, that child will grow up to be unhealthy and probably unhappy, too.

For your child's well-being, save those chips and cookies for what my family refers to as a "blue moon treat," meaning an indulgence that we reserve for special occasions—when we're on vacation or in the company of family and friends. Don't forbid your child from ever tak-ing a bite of junk food— Jean-Pierre Barral put it best when he wrote: "Parents who know how to explain and give good advice don't need to forbid." Talk to your kids about why eating junk food is bad, so that by the time they're adolescents, they're educated enough to make healthy decisions even when you're not around.

This is how we're raising Wyatt—it's not as if we never, ever permit potato chips to cross the threshold of our kitchen. Not at all; absolute denial is never a good idea. We do keep chips in our house, but instead of munching them thoughtlessly every day of the week, we save them for a treat—once a month, or every other weekend on a Saturday night, or during a Sunday ball game. Ordering in a pizza, or eating out in a restaurant, also counts as a blue moon treat. The rest of the time, we stick to a healthy, whole food, organic, vegan diet.

Instilling these healthy eating habits in our kids is so, so important—I really can't emphasize it enough. These lessons, if conveyed early on, will endure long into adulthood. If you give your child healthy food and explain your reasons for doing so, I predict he won't want more than the occasional slice of pizza, or candy bar, or whatever his favorite blue-moon indulgence might be. Turn to the page 240 of resources section for my family's favorite blue moon treats.

Chapter 7

Infancy and Early Childhood

Since the very first months of Wyatt's life, I've filled almost a dozen notebooks with observations about his eating habits and daily activities. After jotting down the date and location, I list everything he ate during the day, as well as any special events, like birthdays or other celebrations, that might have taken place.

I recommend that you adopt the same practice at the very beginning of your child's life—you might be amazed by what you'll learn over the years. Spend just five minutes at the end of every day jotting down notes about your kids. As your child grows older and more independent, you'll find these journals extremely valuable, particularly if your child's behavior or health changes unexpectedly. For example, when Wyatt was two, he seemed to be allergic to something. By referring back to my journal, I could track what exactly he'd been eating when he had these allergic reactions. Thanks to the notes, we quickly confirmed that he was allergic to cantaloupe and eggs at the time.

Keeping a diary also allows you to reflect on the big picture of your child's development. By glancing over your notes, you can determine whether your child really is getting a balanced, healthy diet rich in fruits, veggies, whole grains, nuts, and seeds. You'll be surprised by how this journal helps to keep your child on the right track.

In the years to come, when your kids get old enough, they can help you take notes—by writing down what they ate at school, how they felt about their days, and that sort of thing. In fact, even before they've learned to write, kids can talk to you about their daily experiences. These brief daily reflections will play a big role in helping you understand your child.

Playtime: Rethinking Your Toy Philosophy

We want our children's toys to be fun, safe, and educational. Unfortunately, many popular toys on the market are made with plastic polyvinyl chloride (known as PVC or vinyl) and phthalates, which soften PVC plastic. Some toys imported from China and other countries have been found to be contaminated with lead paint. When you're shopping for toys, be sure to check the country where they were made. In recent years, and even more so after last summer's lead scare, toy stores have actually started to categorize their merchandise by country of origin, because not all countries have the same product safety standards.

But there are other less concrete considerations you should also take into account when choosing your children's toys. Try to shift your emphasis from quantity to quality. Kids don't need a million different toys to keep their imaginations occupied. Rather than cluttering your child's room with tons of cheap plastic toys, why not choose a few elegantly crafted, high-quality toys instead? They will last longer and fuel your child's imagination to higher levels. When I was a toddler, my most prized possession was a wooden Fisher-Price bumblebee that I dragged everywhere with me on a little string. (Toddlers love pull toys; as soon as they learn to walk, they're eager to drag something behind them.) There was nothing high tech or flashy about this toy, but I loved it above all others, and I still have it!

All objects have energy, and the toys our kids play with help form their tastes and preferences. Toys can either teach our kids that objects are disposable or that they are worth valuing and treasuring. Because he never played with throwaway toys as a young child, Wyatt has never been attracted to the latest must-have trendy toys; he doesn't even ask for them. The same is true for electronics equipment. Wyatt has never had a Game Boy, or an Xbox, or any other video-game player. When kids at the ranch find out that he doesn't know how to play video games, they feel sorry for him! Kids today get enough media stimulation without our introducing more into their leisure hours.

Even after Wyatt outgrew his toys, he still liked having them around, and to this day we keep them in his room as architectural pieces. A nice collection of wooden toys will last generations, and when your kids start their own families, they can pass along their favorite toys to their children. When I was growing up, my friend next door to me had this beautiful wooden dollhouse, and we would spend hours playing with it. She still has that dollhouse, and it still looks just as wonderful and magical as it ever did. Can you imagine a plastic toy today lasting that long?

Purchasing Environmentally Friendly Toys

The risk of exposure to toxic substances is particularly high for infants and young children, who tend to put toys in their mouths. Luckily, you can take just a few simple precautions to protect your child from hazardous toys:

Make sure your kids' toys are lead free: Lead, like so many heavy metals, is a highly toxic substance that's especially harmful to children under six years old. Ranked the number-one environmental health threat to young children, lead can be harmful even in small amounts. While the main sources of lead exposure are paint dust and old pipes, many children today are coming into contact with this lethal neurotoxin—which has been linked to reduced IQ, learning disabilities, and behavioral and attention disorders—through their toys.

Yes, that's right—toys are a major route of lead exposure. Though lead paint has been banned since 1978, and lead piping since 1986, there is currently no law mandating that children's toys be free of this fatal poison (unless they have lead paint on them, in which case the lead paint law applies). As demonstrated by the unprecedented recall of millions of Chinese-made toys last year, many children's toys manufactured abroad still contain appalling quantities of lead. Until the Lead Free Toys Act becomes law, parents must be very careful when choosing the toys they bring into their homes. All of the following items might contain lead:

Costume or play jewelry, especially items made of metal, plastic cords, and fake pearls

Metal charms and toy trinkets

Vinyl lunch boxes or other toys imported from China. According to Reuters, a "2005 report in a Beijing newspaper cited estimates that 60 percent of Chinese-made toys used paint with lead above internationally accepted limits."

Painted toys (some, especially those made in China, could be covered in lead paint)

Toy trains

Vinyl bibs

Vinyl backpacks

Jackets with lead buttons or zippers

And bear in mind that hand-to-mouth contact with contaminated substances increases the dangers of lead, which is why experts worry more about lead trinkets than lead lunchboxes: Children are much more likely to put the smaller items in their mouths.

Other possible sources of lead contamination include:

Keys

Lead sinkers for fishing

Lead soldiers and other collectible figurines

Colored newsprint, including comic books

Colored food wrappers with ink printed on plastic bags; don't reuse these

Older ceramic dishes and imported dishes

Imported eyeliner and face paint for children

Because all of the health problems associated with lead exposure are totally preventable, it's really important to take an inventory of your home. If you turn up any of the above suspect items, you can easily check them with an inexpensive do-it-yourself lead-test kit that's available at hardware stores for about twenty dollars. (You can find these kits on the Internet as well, at sites like www.leadinspector.com, www.leadcheck.com, and www.leadtesttoys.com.) While extremely easy to use, these lead-testing strips or swabs can on occasion produce inaccurate results, and they do not indicate the amount of lead present in an item. You should also check the Web site of the U.S. Consumer Product Safety Commission (www.cpsc.gov) for important recall information on specific toys.

Until toys containing lead have been banned from this country, you might want to consider getting your child tested for lead. Recommendations vary state by state—in New Jersey, children are tested at ages one and two—but I think yearly testing through early adolescence is a good idea. Following the recent lead-toys scare, some parents are asking for tests every three to six months for children under the age of five.

For more information and resources, visit www.leadsafenj.org.

The Lessons of Lead

While we still have an enormous amount to learn about how chemicals influence children's health, everything we do know "started with lead," said Dr. Phil Landrigan. "Lead has caused so much disease and so much misery in kids in this country and around the world. But what we learned from lead is that children are more vulnerable than adults, that much lower levels of poison can cause damage in them, compared with adults. We learned that the damage that lead causes is like an iceberg. So at the tip of the iceberg you have the very obvious lead poisoning in children who are exposed to high doses, that results in kids who come into the emergency room with pulmonary convulsions. But we also learned that at lower levels lead is also toxic, that it can cause brain damage, that it can reduce children's IQ, that it can mess up their behavior, that it can shorten their attention span, can increase the risk that they're going to drop out of high school, increase the risk that they're going to end up in prison. And all of those lessons that we learned from lead, we've now applied to a whole series of other substances."

Given these horrifying "lessons," we might assume that lead is a "solved issue," as Dr. Landrigan put it. Unfortunately, that's far from being the case. "We've progressed a great deal," he said, "but we still have a lot to do. The CDC numbers show that we've reduced the incidence of lead poisoning by 90 percent, and the average blood lead level in American kids by slightly more than 90 percent. The problem is," he went on, "we still have thousands of housing units in the United States that have lead paint. Every year, we have new cases of lead poisoning."

Nurse Barbara McGoey agreed. "Lead levels are still atrocious with children in our country," she said. "And it's not because they're sitting around eating paint chips, but because of the environment they're living in. Lead's in their water, their toys, the dust in the air from the buses. It's just everywhere. We've had kids with bad, bad lead levels." If lead is such a problem, why don't we test our kids' levels more thoroughly? At the moment, we only test kids at the ages of one and two, even though some aren't contaminated until later in life.

This protocol must change. You can determine lead levels with a simple finger-prick test, so why aren't we testing kids every year, up to the age of fifteen? If a child does have lead poisoning, it's necessary to chelate, or undergo an elaborate treatment that uses chemicals to pull certain toxic metals out of the body. The sooner doctors discover the elevated lead levels, the better their chances of minimizing the damage.

The CDC now estimates that three hundred thousand children between the ages of one and five in the United

States have "unsafe" levels of lead in their blood. The CDC defines the threshold of "safe" blood-lead levels at 10 micrograms per deciliter. Inner-city children in particular have disproportionately high levels of lead in their blood. The prevalence of elevated blood-lead levels among African-American children living in large inner cities is around 36 percent, while the prevalence among higher-income white suburban children is around 4 percent.

"People tend to think of lead poisoning as a disease of poor children," said Dr. Landrigan. "And that is true in 85 percent of kids; it's kids who live in old, dilapidated, mostly urban housing. But that still leaves 15 percent of the cases that occur in middle- or upper-class families, usually associated with home renovations. People are sanding paint, removing banisters, cleaning up windowsills, and they don't realize that they're spewing lead dust around in the house. And then the kids get it. So we have a campaign that we've been trying to organize through hardware stores and other stores that cater to the do-it-yourselfer, to warn people of the hazards of deleading."

And bear in mind that paint isn't the only issue. Pre-1980s plumbing systems may also contain lead, so consider having your home water checked for lead as well. Always use a water filter and be sure to use only cold water for cooking and drinking.

Frequent (but not obsessive) hand washing provides a reliable shield from all sorts of contamination, including infectous agents and toxins. "Parents should always be very aware of having kids wash their hands before they eat," said Dr. Kenneth Bock. "And if either parent works in an industry that exposes them to some kinds of toxins, make sure they change before they come home, meaning they take off their work clothes before they hug the kids as well as washing the work clothes separately—not with the kids' stuff."

If you're still worried about lead residues, there are other common-sense measures you can take to protect your kids. Wash your child's hands, face, bottles, pacifiers, and toys often. Wet mop or wipe down hard surfaces frequently, especially floors and windowsills, to remove any traces of lead dust. Use only cold water for drinking and cooking. And if it's a possibility for you, have a certified professional test lead levels in your house.

Make sure your kids' toys are PVC free. PVC, or polyvinyl chloride or vinyl, is widely considered the most damaging plastic for human health and the environment. This chlorine byproduct is used as a raw material in the manufacture of a huge number of consumer products: plastic water bottles, vinyl flooring, shower curtains, as well as pacifiers and children's toys. Young children, who are apt to suck or chew on their toys, are particularly susceptible to PVC exposure. Many European countries have already banned the use of PVCs in baby toys, but this battle hasn't yet been won in the United States. The good news is, with just a little effort, you can make sure that your children's toys are free of these potentially harmful chemicals. When shopping for baby products, look for labels marked "No PVCs." For more information on the dangers of PVC, refer to www.checnet.org/healthehouse/education/articles-detail.asp?Main_ID=185.

Make sure your kids' toys are phthalate free.
Phthalates are used in everything from cosmetics to plastic PVC toys. These potentially dangerous toxins, which make PVC plastics soft and pliable, have been linked to kidney and liver damage, as well as endocrine disruption. Because phthalates are used to soften plastics, they are traditionally used in teething rings and other chew toys for babies, as well as beach balls and bath toys for older children. (In general, the stiffer and harder the toy is, the less likely it is to contain phthalates.)

Diisononyl phthalate (DINP), the most commonly used phthalate in soft plastic vinyl children's toys, has been shown to cause liver and kidney damage and cancer in laboratory animals. The government does not require inclusion of phthalates on ingredient lists. As a general rule, I recommend that you avoid teethers, pacifiers, and other soft plastic toys that are not specifically labeled "phthalate free." Be particularly careful with a vinyl toy that is ripped or torn, since the tear is where the phthalates are most likely to escape. For more information on phthalates, please visit www.mindfully.org/Plastic/Plasticizers/About-Phthalates .htm.

Whenever possible, opt for wooden toys with nontoxic finishes. Wooden toys reduce the demand for plastic-made versions and the toxic chemicals used in their production. Just make sure those toys have nontoxic finishes.

Make sure your kids' toys contain no formaldehyde.
Formaldehyde, a known carcinogen, is used in everything from wrinkle-free fabric finishes to some adhesives. It is

commonly used in the glues of engineered wood (such as plywood) and MDF (medium-density fiberboard) products.

Give your kids toys that don't require batteries. Toys powered by a child's imagination are often more educational and allow for more imaginative play than battery-powered toys. Battery-free toys also reduce the demand for the toxic components used in battery production and the burden put on the waste stream when they have run out.

Buy toys that have been made in the U.S.A. Buying domestically manufactured toys has several benefits: it supports jobs and local economies, and it also reduces the fossil fuels needed to ship items. Environmental standards are also often higher here than in countries such as China.

Wyatt's Favorite Toys

Wyatt always loved Waldorf dolls—and yes, boys should play with dolls, too. I believe playing with dolls sets a solid foundation of caretaking that will prepare Wyatt for fatherhood. Now that he's nine years old, he has a very nurturing attitude toward all the kids with cancer who come to the ranch in New Mexico.

From the age of one, Wyatt played constantly with his Waldorf dolls—he could spend all day playing house and taking care of his babies. He picked each one out himself, every one a different race, with different colored hair. We still have these dolls and will keep them forever—they are family heirlooms.

We found his favorite handmade Waldorf dolls at Magic Cabin (www.magiccabin.com), which is one of the absolute best toymakers around. Their fair-trade toys are all extremely imaginative and beautifully crafted. Magic Cabin also offers a great variety of different toys for babies and toddlers alike. Their catalog is wonderful, with housekeeping sets, wooden tree houses, and puzzles.

Willow Tree Toys (www.willowtreetoys.com) also makes gorgeous fair-trade Waldorf dolls. Three Sisters Toys (www.threesisterstoys.com) sells wonderful playstands made out of untreated wood. A child can play all day long at a playstand, relying entirely on her imagination. Three Sisters also sells accessories to go in or around the playstands: silk rainbow blankets and scapes. You can also find cherrywood rattles, amber teething necklaces, wooden picture books, and mobiles. Wyatt still has the Nils Holgersson book and mobile hanging in his bedroom.

We found most of Wyatt's other favorite toys at North Star Toys (www.northstartoys.com). North Star is a fantastic family-run business that makes all their toys by hand. Everything is wooden, nontoxic, and beautiful. Wyatt loved the wooden farm set, the wooden magic wands, and their brilliant wooden puzzles. I particularly recommend North Star's great selection of wooden puzzles for kids between the ages of two and seven—they make ideal gifts.

Hazelnut Kids (www.hazelnutkids.com) sold our favorite art supplies. We particularly love the chunky nontoxic beeswax crayons made by the German company Stockmar. Stockmar also makes colored pencils, watercolor paints, block beeswax crayons, and modeling beeswax. When Wyatt was five, the two of us created an entire winter scene from modeling beeswax. We worked on it for an entire week, and every winter, we still display it in our house. Lyra is another great art-supply brand sold by Hazelnut Kids, Waldorf Toys, and Magic Cabin. Lyra makes beautiful colored pencils and kits that Wyatt loves. For more extensive resources on environmentally friendly toys, including art supplies, please see page 259 in the resources section.

Bathing Your Baby

Bathing children is, for many families, a cherished end-of-day ritual. Just make sure that you know exactly what you're putting in your child's bath. After all, the skin is the largest organ of the body, and some of the most acute chemical exposures are transmitted through dermal contact.

Recent laboratory tests released by environmental author David Steinman and the nonprofit Campaign for Safe Cosmetics found 1,4-dioxane in a range of children's bath washes and bubble baths. The EPA lists 1,4-dioxane as a probable human carcinogen, while the National Toxicology Program recognizes it as an animal carcinogen.

Most parents and caregivers are unaware that the FDA does not require safety testing on cosmetics before they are sold to the public, which means that manufacturers can legally sell many products containing a cocktail of unproven, potentially unsafe chemicals. Thousands of these products are marketed to children. For a listing of the products tested, and the amounts of 1,4-dioxane found in each, visit: www.ewg .org/issues_content/cosmetics/pdf/14-dioxane.pdf.

For healthier alternatives for your baby, natural and organic products are available at many major food stores and mass merchandisers, as well as health food stores. But be careful: 1,4 dioxane does not need to be listed among a product's ingredients (because it is a byproduct of manufacturing, not an additive) and it may be present even in some so-called "natural" products made by major retailers. For more information on these issues, see the Environmental Working Group's coverage (www.safecosmetics.org/newsroom/press.cfm?pressReleaseID-21).

Choose brands such as Aubrey Organics or Earth's Best to avoid unnecessary chemicals. California Baby (www.californiababy.com) and Weleda (www.usa.weleda.com) also make great organic personal-care products for babies. A great alternative to traditional baby shampoo is

Jason *Kids Only!* Shampoo, which contains no SLS (sodium lauryl sulfate). Some other bathing guidelines:

- Use 100 percent natural products, unscented, dye free, packaged in recycled or recyclable packaging. Make sure soaps contain no synthetic chemicals.

- Buy products with the least amount of packaging to reduce unnecessary waste.

- Buy products with the least amount of packaging to reduce unnecessary waste.

- Avoid any petroleum-based/mineral oil–based formulas.

- Avoid any product with "fragrance," which could refer to any combination of unspecified chemicals, including phthalates.

- Talk to your pediatrician about alternatives to conventional fluoridated toothpaste, as recent research has caused scientists to question the benefits of fluoride in the public water system. Fluoride might be both ineffective and dangerous, linked to health effects as serious as a rare bone cancer in boys; for more information on this ongoing debate, visit the Fluoride Action Network (www .fluoridealert.org). As a safe alternative, we like Jason organics for Wyatt.

And for babies, I recommend getting a Tummy Tub from the New Zealand company Nature Baby (www.naturebaby.co.nz). It's the very best baby bathtub you can buy—deep and upright to give your baby the secure feeling of being inside the womb. The unique shape also prevents your baby from sliding.

Other Bathing Tips:

As I mention earlier, the tap water in our homes might be contaminated with any number of toxins, and we aren't just exposed by drinking the water—contact through bathing and showering is another concern. If you can't install a water-filtration system in your home (see page 258), you can still easily cut down on the toxins in your water: reduce the harmful effects of many of the toxins that might be in your water:

- Brush the skin before bathing and showering. You can find a body brush in health food stores and even most conventional drugstores. Brushing the skin stimulates circulation and helps to open pores to eliminate toxins. You can massage and brush toddlers, too, as long as you're extremely gentle. For babies, a little massage before bathtime serves a similar purpose.

- Sea salt baths are wonderful detoxifiers. You can buy solar sea salt rocks in health food stores. Brenda Brock's Farmaesthetics (www.farmaesthetics.com) and Susan Ciminelli (www.susanciminelli.com) both make wonderful solar sea salts, with sprigs of lavender and other healing, relaxing essential oils added.

- Apple cider vinegar baths (see opposite) are both detoxifying and extremely relaxing.

- When bathing babies, toddlers, and young children, always keep the doors and windows of the bathroom wide open. You don't want your kids breathing in the chlorine vapors from the steam.

The Benefits of Apple Cider Vinegar

From the time he was three years old, I've poured half a cup of apple cider vinegar into Wyatt's bath. Apple cider vinegar is extremely therapeutic. It's not only a great cleanser and detoxifier, but it also provides a number of different health benefits, like boosting children's moods and helping them relax.

Wyatt has faced a lot of emotional ups and downs throughout his years at the ranch. Many kids who've become his friends have later died of cancer, which has been devastating for him. Taking long baths has helped him relax and deal with his emotions. And last summer, we adopted a shelter dog that followed Wyatt around every second. Even though he knows they'll be reunited next summer, Wyatt was heartbroken to leave that dog behind at the end of the summer. When we got back to New York, he was feeling a little deflated, and he said to me, "Mom, I just need a long soak in apple cider vinegar."

Apple cider vinegar can also make bathtime a lot more fun. When mixed with bubble bath (our family favorite is California Baby), vinegar produces thick foam and amazing, two-foot-high bubbles that kids love. Wyatt and I discovered this trick completely by accident one day—I'd poured in the cider vinegar as usual, and then just for fun we added some bubbles.

Relaxation Techniques

Infant massage is a wonderful way to help both babies and mothers relax. You can buy a guidebook to infant massage, or you can just do whatever feels natural and therapeutic to you. Use therapeutic-grade essential oils (see page 254) for additional efficacy. On Wyatt, I used lavender to help him relax and get to sleep. Of course, you should always check with your doctor before using any essential oils. There are some oils that you should avoid during pregnancy and others your baby should avoid.

Reiki is another great technique for helping both babies and mommies relax. This ancient Japanese healing art uses hands-on touch to reduce stress and promote relaxation. When Wyatt was younger, I taught him a few Reiki techniques that he practices whenever he's feeling fearful, confused, or anxious. Just a little Reiki instruction has helped Wyatt become more centered and relaxed. Turn to the resources section for my recommendations on infant-massage and Reiki books.

Teething Tools

I know that teething can be painful for babies, but don't fall prey to the temptation to buy your child a plastic teething toy. Plastics containing PVCs, phthalates, and other toxins are the very last things I would want my child putting into his mouth! Instead, I recommend an amber teething necklace, which you can purchase at Nova Natural Toys and Crafts (www.novanatural.com). But do be aware that babies should under *no* circumstances chew on these amber necklaces—their soothing benefits come from contact with the baby's skin. If you do decide to get your child an amber necklace, you must make absolutely sure that the necklace is too short for your child to put in his mouth. The beads should also be individually knotted, so that there's no danger of beads spilling all over the floor. Another safe option is the Under the Nile organic cotton bumblebee teething ring that you can buy at Hazelnut Kids (www.hazelnutkids.com). You can also try some homeopathic remedies from Hylands and Boiron. Rubbing your baby's gums is also effective, but I absolutely don't recommend rubbing them with any quantity of brandy or any other alcohol.

The Diaper Dilemma

Diapers present some tough issues for a parent committed to protecting the environment. With Wyatt, I first tried cloth cotton diapers. I bought all these beautiful organic cotton diapers and then almost immediately encountered a problem: Where could I get them washed? Every single laundry service I contacted used heavy-duty toxins, like chlorine bleach, to wash the diapers. To me, this seemed to defeat the whole purpose of having organic cotton. So, for about four months, I washed all of the diapers myself, but pretty soon, I became completely overwhelmed by this task—there I was, with a newborn, washing at least ten diapers every day!

Even with help, I couldn't keep up, so eventually I started alternating between the cloth diapers and Tushies chlorine-bleach-free disposable diapers. Tushies (www.tushies.com) makes good disposable diapers and wipes without chlorine bleach, perfumes, dyes, or artificial chemical absorbents like the acid polymer salts used by the leading brands. These healthier disposables are widely available at Wild Oats, Whole Foods, and other leading health-food stores.

Obviously, no disposable is ideal, but these brands are a lot healthier than traditional diapers, which can leach out toxins. Try alternating between these toxin-free disposables and cloth diapers, like the all-in-ones sold at ClothDiaper.com, which offer "the convenience of a disposable in a reusable cloth diaper" at competitive prices.

I'd also stay away from those rubber pants that some parents put on over the diaper for extra protection. Do you really want to encase your child in rubber and create a compost pile out of your baby's poop? It's just not healthy—it's like putting a plastic bag around your baby.

I had another diaper dilemma several years later, when Wyatt was a toddler and too big for regular diapers but not yet completely potty trained. What could I use? The "pull-ups" that are made out of diaper material but designed to resemble underwear are the most obvious choice, but unfortunately, Tushies and other eco-friendly companies didn't yet make a pull-up. In the end, I had no choice but to use the traditional (i.e., toxic) pull-up brands for an entire year, which was very, very upsetting for me.

I prefer the cloth alternatives by Kushies (www.kushies.com), which makes healthy cloth diapers and pull-ups for toddlers, as well as organic changing pads, layettes, and baby clothes. Cloth pull-ups are much less expensive than disposables and better for the environment as well. Another advantage: the experience of having an accident usually inspires kids to train faster. Because disposable pull-ups are so heavily advertised, most parents don't realize this alternative exists, but I'd recommend looking into it.

To treat diaper rash, avoid talcum powder, which can cause serious respiratory problems if inhaled by a baby. Yes, it does a great job of absorbing moisture, but it has also been linked to cancer in some animal studies—do you really want your baby to come into contact with such a substance? A healthier alternative is arrowroot powder—that's what I used when Wyatt was a baby. I also used calendula cream on his bottom to prevent diaper rash. Weleda and Jurlique both make great calendula creams.

Lis Youhanic from Fort Mill, South Carolina, wrote me with another suggestion:

> *I was surprised to find out while talking with family and friends*
> *how few of them know about using cornstarch for diaper*

rashes on their babies. Please let your readers know that they can use cornstarch with nothing else in it just like they would baby powder and I have found that it not only prevents rashes from recurring but helped my son heal from his—and he has extremely sensitive skin, so finding products he can use is tricky, but the cornstarch worked every time! And since the powder isn't as fine as baby powder, I didn't worry about him breathing it in and irritating his lungs.

Sun Protection

Very early in life, you and your child should get into the habit of protecting his skin from the sun—not just on rare excursions to the beach, but every single day of the year, even in the dead of winter. However nice the sun feels warming your shoulders, overexposure to ultraviolet (UV) radiation can have serious adverse health effects over the long term. Children overexposed to the sun might not experience these effects—which include skin cancer, prematurely aged skin, and eye damage—until much later in life, which is all the more reason to prevent the damage from ever occurring. The thinning of the ozone layer leaves kids today more vulnerable than ever to UV radiation.

The Environmental Protection Agency has developed an educational program (available on the Web at www.epa.gov/sunwise) to teach kids about how to protect themselves from harmful UV radiation. The EPA SunWise program also lists these common-sense "action steps" kids (and their parents) can take to minimize exposure:

- Stay out of the sun in the middle of the day. The sun's rays are strongest between the hours of 10:00 a.m. and 4:00 p.m. If you are outside during those hours, retire to the shade for as long as you can.

- Always wear a wide-brimmed hat when outdoors for an extended period of time.

- Choose sunglasses that protect from UV radiation to prevent eye damage.

- Avoid sunlamps and tanning parlors.

- Wear long sleeves. Loose-fitting clothing of tightly knit fabrics provides some sun protection.

- *Always, always* wear a broad-spectrum sunblock with a sun protection factor (SPF) of 15 or greater. When exercising, swimming, or outdoors for an extended period of time, reapply frequently, at least every two hours.

It's important to find a sunscreen that protects you from both UVA and UVB rays, because while UVB rays cause sunburn, UVA ray penetrate the skin deeper and might cause more serious damage over time. UVA rays also intensify the cancer-causing effects of UVB rays.

Finding a truly nontoxic sunscreen can be extremely challenging. But as a general rule, sunblocks (which physically "block" the sun's rays) contain fewer potentially harmful chemicals than sunscreens (which chemically absorb the rays). Look for a sunblock containing minerals like zinc dioxide or titanium dioxide, which don't penetrate the skin. For recommendations on safe, effective sunblocks, please refer to the resources section.

The Pet Question

For many of us, a family doesn't feel complete without a pet, or several pets—I know our Norfolk terrier, Virgil, is a VIP in our household. Pets can be great for children: they're great both for companionship and for teaching kids responsibility. More and more of us welcome domestic animals into our homes every year: At last count, Americans owned an estimated 90.5 million cats and 73.9 million dogs.

Always make sure that your pets—and your children—are as safe as possible. If you own a cat, you should definitely consult your doctor about the possibility of contracting toxoplasmosis, which can cause serious birth defects, during pregnancy. (As long as you stay away from the litter box, it's extremely unlikely that your cat will transmit the disease to you.) But toxoplasmosis isn't the only consideration you need to take into account when combining kids and pets. Many of the pet-care products that we use can be dangerous to the health of not only our pets, but of our children as well.

The already huge pet-care industry is growing bigger—and more powerful—every year. In 2004, we spent $34.4 billion dollars on pet-care products, almost twice what we spent just a decade earlier. Every year, we buy more and more specialty items for our pets, most of which our furry critters neither want nor need.

Our pets are far more vulnerable to chemical exposures than we are. Cats and many dogs, like young children, are small in size and travel close to the ground. Indoors, they're more likely to come into contact with the toxins in conventional cleaning products; outdoors, with toxic gases, bacteria, and other hazardous particulate matter.

So rather than increase your pets' chemical burden by washing them with toxic shampoos and placing carcinogenic flea collars around their necks, you need to work on reducing that burden. Never, ever take your pet to a groomer or vet who uses toxic grooming products, because you're not just poisoning your pet; you're poisoning your child as well. Think about what happens when you bring your clean, fluffy pet home in the evening. Your kids will probably fall all over their beloved friend, hugging and kissing it, rubbing their faces into the animal's fur and breathing in all those toxins from the chemical shampoos.

Ask your groomer to stop using toxic products on your pet. If he refuses, find another groomer. Or better yet, just bathe your animal at home. Don't think of it as a chore, but as a fun project that the whole family can conquer as a team.

When I shampoo our dog Virgil, I use the same organic shampoos that my son and husband and I use on our own hair: Avalon Organics, Aubrey Organics, or John Masters Organics. These great-smelling, healthy products all contain essential oils with a number of useful properties. For Virgil and our other dogs at the ranch, I especially like the formulas that contain ylang-ylang, which is a natural bug repellant. Other pest-deterring shampoo ingredients include sage, lemongrass, eucalyptus, and rosemary.

Which brings us to another major issue: flea prevention. Even if your pet has a serious flea problem, you should never, ever put a toxic flea collar around his neck. Children who grow up with dogs who wear toxic flea collars have a dramatically higher incidence of brain tumors and other cancers. Every time your kids pet the dog, they're soaking those dangerous pesticides—which include organophosphates and carbamate compounds—right up. And just think what they're doing to your pet!

And most of the time, flea collars don't even work that well. You'll do a better job of preventing fleas by taking these simple precautions:

- Wash your pet on a regular basis with nontoxic soap and water.

- Vacuum your home frequently and thoroughly during flea season to get rid of any flea eggs.

- Wash your animal's bedding as often as you do your own.

- To keep fleas off our dogs at the ranch, we mix a little brewer's yeast powder into our dogs' food bowl every morning, which makes the animals less attractive to fleas, flies, and other pests. You could also try administering the brewer's yeast in a tablet—dogs don't seem to mind the taste.

- Add garlic to your dogs' diets. You can put garlic in either a dehydrated powder or flake form directly onto the dogs' food, or you can wrap up a pill in a little piece of soy cheese.

These two supplements—brewer's yeast and garlic—not only repel fleas; they add shine to your dogs' coats and boost their immune systems. Essential oils can also help: putting some eucalyptus near your pets' sleeping area will also work to fend off the fleas. If you still want to try a flea collar, there are several companies that make nontoxic plant-and-essential-oil-based flea collars that fight off fleas without damaging your animal—or child—in the process. Only Natural Pet (www.onlynaturalpet.com) and Holistic Family and Pets (www .holisticfamilyandpets.com) both have several different flea- and tick-collar options. Only Natural Pet also has a great selection of high-quality nontoxic pet foods, cat litter, grooming products, dietary supplements, and accessories.

But in general, you don't need to spend a lot of money keeping your pet happy and healthy. A nourishing diet and plenty of love usually do the trick.

Chapter 8

Green Pediatrics

In recent years, we've seen a new and exciting movement in the field of medicine, especially pediatric medicine: the emergence of the "green" doctor. Green pediatricians promote what Dr. Lawrence Rosen calls "a philosophy of whole child care."

Children, he said, are "not just physical beings. They are made up of a mind, a body, and a spirit that all come together." Accordingly, green pediatricians like Dr. Rosen believe that children's "health is dependent on not just their physical biochemical state, but also on how they interact with their parents, their family, their community at large, the environment they live in. And those systems all have an impact on what we call the child's health."

Dr. Rosen went on to emphasize a core practice of green doctors. "Integrative pediatricians," he said, "believe that prevention is better than treatment after the fact. We also believe that using the body's own natural resources is more powerful, and often more effective, than using very specific targeted conventional medications." There are, Dr. Rosen said, no quick fixes in green medicine, no magic pills that take effect overnight.

Some integrative pediatricians are searching for healthier ways to treat the symptoms of even the most serious childhood illnesses, like cancer. Integrative pediatric oncologist Susan Sencer describes her field both as both "high tech" (meaning it requires access to the latest technology) and "high touch" (meaning it involves a personal, holistic approach that differs from child to child).

In Minneapolis, Sencer and her coworkers use a variety of mind-body therapies to improve the quality of life of kids with cancer, including hypnosis, massage, acupuncture, and biofeedback. "Pediatric medicine has always been more holistic than adult medicine," Sencer told me. "The higher up we get on the specialty food chain in adult medicine, the more we lose touch with the big picture."

In other areas, too, green medicine has enjoyed a growing popularity in the field of pediatrics. At Hackensack, with the help of dedicated practitioners like Dr. Rosen and nurse Karen Overgaard, we are energetically exploring the healing potential of alternative modalities like hypnosis, Reiki, massage, and acupuncture. We're also working to bring more green doctors and nurses into mainstream medical practices, general hospitals, and teaching hospitals across the country.

In our search for healthier, more holistic ways to take care of our children, we're placing a greater emphasis on diet and nutrition as well. In this particular respect, we have a long way to go. Just look at the food served in typical hospitals: artificially processed, high in additives, salt, sugar and artificial sweeteners, and trans fatty acids. We already know how important a healthy whole-foods diet is in maintaining our kids' health. So why are we feeding kids who are already sick food that does nothing to heal their ailing bodies? If anything, this food only creates *more* problems.

Dr. Sencer's integrative oncology center has established many nutritional holistic protocols for kids with cancer. "Some kids are so micronutrient poor," she said, "that I recommend everyone take a vitamin. For kids, though, it's very hard to make dietary changes when they've just been diagnosed with cancer, or when they're going through chemotherapy. The high doses of steroids make people crave foods high in sodium—Big Macs, fries, that sort of thing. They'll crave something familiar and comforting, and unfortunately for most of them that's what McDonald's is."

But all too often, these "comfort foods" only make the problem worse. "Obesity," Sencer said, "is coming to dwarf cancer as a childhood health problem, and this is a huge concern, since obesity sets kids up for just about every adult health problem you can think of later in life. If we could improve one thing across the board," she went on, "I'd pick nutrition. Nutrition is really our biggest problem in this country." She said point blank that "the fact that most doctors don't talk about nutrition with their patients is sinful."

As green pediatricians like Sencer become more common, we're hoping to see more discussions along these lines—discussions about nutrition and lifestyle that can make a crucial difference in the future health of a child. Today, integrative pediatricians are still a minority, but I predict that one day not too far in the future, they'll enter the mainstream of pediatric medicine. And when that happens, our kids will benefit across the board.

Vaccinations: Medicine's Greatest Achievement or Too Much of a Good Thing?

In this section, I want to talk to you candidly about what is likely to be your baby's first, and perhaps most important, medical intervention: vaccinations. It's important for you to get as much information about vaccines as possible so you can make an informed choice about what's best for your baby. The following pages address some issues that you are unlikely to hear speaking with your pediatrician, and they have been the source of much debate. It is important for you to get as much information about vaccines as possible so you can decide what's best for *your* baby.

Parents must understand both the benefits and risks associated with vaccines. The benefits are obvious: Vaccinations create immunity to diseases by inducing the body to make antibodies against diseases. They play a critical role in preventing serious illnesses and infectious diseases.

From a public-health standpoint, vaccines are essential in maintaining what is called "herd immunity," meaning that they help to protect the public as a whole. In other words, your child is vaccinated first and foremost to protect the "herd."

The Centers for Disease Control and Prevention (CDC) has estimated that we vaccinate approximately 80 percent of our population, a practice that has greatly reduced the spread of many harmful infectious diseases in our society. Take measles as an example: Before the introduction of the measles vaccine in the United States, there were approximately five hundred thousand reported cases and five hundred deaths annually from the disease. In 1998, there were only one hundred reported cases of measles in the United States. No one can deny that's a dramatic improvement.

So what could possibly be the drawbacks of vaccinations?

There has always been some controversy surrounding this subject, and like all controversies, this one has two sides. One side is easy to find on television and in newspaper articles. There's no shortage of stories about new vaccines and warnings about the "dire" consequences people will face if they don't vaccinate their children. The other side is rarely reported and takes a little time and research to understand.

Because vaccines are considered medicine's "greatest lifesaver," credited with eradicating many contagious diseases, more and more vaccines have been developed and added to the recommended immunization schedule over the past twenty years. When I was growing up, we received only six vaccines. Today's current generation of children receive on average forty-nine doses of fourteen vaccines before the age of six. Compare the difference:

CDC Recommended Immunization Schedule Comparison

Birth to 6 years

1983		2007	
Vaccine	**Month administered**	**Vaccine**	**Month administered**
DTP*	2	Influenza	prenatal
OPV	2	Hep B	birth
DTP*	4	Hep B	1
OPV	4	DTaP*	2
DTP*	6	Hib	2
MMR*	15	IPV	2
DTP*	18	PCV	2
OPV	18	Rotavirus	2
		Hep B	4
		DTaP*	4
		Hib	4
		IPV	4
		PCV	4
		Rotavirus	4
		Hep B	6
		DTaP*	6
		Hib	6
		IPV	6
		PCV	6
		Influenza	6
		Rotavirus	6
		Hib	12
		MMR*	12

1983		2007	
Vaccine	Month administered	Vaccine	Month administered
		Varicella	12
		PCV	12
		Hep A	12
		DTaP*	15
		Hep A	18
		Influenza	18
		Influenza	30
		Influenza	42
		MMR*	48
		DTaP*	48
		IPV	48
		Influenza	54
		Influenza	66
18 Vaccines		50 Vaccines	

*DTP, DTaP, and MMR each contain three vaccines in one shot

To see the complete current recommended childhood vaccine schedule, please refer to www.vaccinesafety.edu/2007-schedule.htm.

If you study this long list of vaccines, you might reasonably assume that America's children, because they are the most vaccinated, are also the healthiest in the world. In reality, the opposite is true: As more and more vaccines have been added to the recommended immunization schedule, the overall health of our children has actually declined. Could there be a connection?

Could the number of vaccines now recommended actually be contributing to the rise in children's chronic diseases like asthma, allergies, autism, autoimmune disease, diabetes, obesity, some cancers, and the growing epidemic of developmental disorders? Remember, in just twenty-four years, we've gone from fewer than ten vaccines to fifty vaccines, and there are more on the way. As the childhood health crisis worsens, more and more parents, and physicians, are starting to question the effect these vaccines might be having on our children's developing immune systems. People are starting to ask themselves, How many vaccines can one little baby handle? Are vaccine manufacturers and the regulatory agencies charged with vaccine safety doing their best to ensure the safety of these vaccines?

Could all of these vaccines be too much of a good thing?

Vaccine Safety Concerns

While it's a terrible tragedy for any child to contract a preventable infectious disease that can result in long-term health complications and even on a very rare occasion death, most children fully recover and then have natural immunity to the disease. It's no less tragic for a child to suffer an avoidable adverse reaction to a vaccine, a reaction that can result in a lifetime of suffering with a chronic and debilitating disease.

Although rarely discussed, adverse reactions are a reality. Some parents would argue that a few hundred cases of measles or chicken pox—diseases that many of us had, and recovered from, in the 1950s—do not justify the suffering of hundreds of thousands of children who may have regressed into autism as a result of the known developmental neurotoxins in many vaccines. These challenging questions require lengthy research and deliberation.

Would it surprise you to know that the majority of parents don't ask any questions about the vaccines given to their babies? Most parents spend more time researching a new car or refrigerator than they will vaccines or vaccine ingredients. We can spend all day searching for the right pair of shoes, but how many of us will devote a full hour to studying the benefits and risks associated with vaccines?

If you were to ask new parents what they know about vaccines and their possible side effects, very few would know that adverse vaccine reactions even exist, much less what to do in the event of one happening, despite having to sign an informal consent form before the vaccination can take place.

Our country's recommended vaccine schedule, which almost all parents follow, fails to take one crucial aspect into account: that every child is different. Some babies—especially ones who are premature, may have had some medical complications or illnesses in the first six months of life, or genetic susceptibility to certain illnesses—may be at an increased risk of experiencing an adverse reaction to certain vaccines.

To minimize these potential risks, we need to work toward more "individualization in the vaccine schedule," suggests Dr. Lawrence Rosen. Our current one-size-fits-all approach to immunizing our children could be placing some vulnerable children at risk to avoidable vaccine reactions, resulting in irreparable harm.

Dr. Kenneth Bock echoes this point, saying that, while he is all for vaccinating children, he thinks that pediatricians should pay closer attention to the needs of each individual case. "When you get into the question of the individual versus public health," he said, "the recommendations for public health may not always be the best for that individual, because of their genetic predisposition and family history of autoimmunity and all that sort of thing." Dr. Bock recommends that we screen our children thoroughly before vaccinating them, to ensure that the inoculations meet their individual needs. We also need to make sure that the vaccines themselves are as safe as possible.

Kids should get vaccinated—of course they should. But while I believe in vaccines, I only vaccinate my son under the following conditions:

- He is not sick or recently recovered from an illness.

- The vaccine must be thimerosal free (see page 135).

- The vaccine should not contain formaldehyde, aluminum, or any other heavy metal. Consult with your doctor about possible alternatives.

- He only receives one vaccine per office visit. If there's not a widespread infectious disease going around, what's the rush?

- The doctor always checks for titers. This means that, after Wyatt is given a vaccine, we check the protective levels of antibodies present in his blood against that agent. To put it another way: A child may have "positive" or "immune" titer levels if either he has been exposed to the infection naturally or if he's been vaccinated. If the results of this simple blood test are positive, indicating immunity, then the child may not need further vaccines of this type.

- The vaccine must be necessary. Most of us had chicken pox when we were children. Given the number of vaccines children already receive, many parents prefer not to give the chicken pox vaccine, often called a "convenience" vaccine, because chicken pox is not considered a life-threatening disease. Some parents prefer to allow their children to develop natural immunity by exposing them to the chicken pox. I choose not to give Wyatt some vaccines if his pediatrician and I conclude that the potential risks outweigh the benefits. Giving Wyatt a vaccine that contains mercury might create far more problems than it solves.

If you have a family history of reactions to any vaccine, or your child has experienced what you believe was a negative reaction to a vaccine in the past, you must absolutely discuss this with your pediatrician and *make sure the reaction is well documented in your child's medical records.* If your child broke out in a rash after taking penicillin, your doctor would be unlikely to give it to him again. The same safety measure should be taken with vaccinations.

There is a saying used by public health agencies: "Be wise—immunize." But there's another saying, too: "Educate before you vaccinate." Making an informed decision about your baby's vaccinations may be one of the most important things you ever do.

Adverse Vaccine Reactions

Because your baby cannot tell you how she feels, you should know how to identify the symptoms of an adverse vaccine reaction. According to the American Academy of Pediatrics' Red Book, "Risks of immunization may vary from trivial and inconvenient to severe and life-threatening." Adverse reactions to vaccines can occur at any age, even in adults, and sometimes weeks after the actual vaccination. Research the new vaccines recommended for your children well in advance and review any new or updated information. Possible adverse reactions to vaccines include:

- **Fever.** While a low fever may be expected, a percentage of children will develop a fever that exceeds 102 degrees Fahrenheit shortly after, or up to twelve days, following vaccination, which can last several days. I recommend that you report any fever your child develops to your physician. If your child's fever falls within the normal range, many physicians do not recommend treating it with Tylenol. "In general, I do not advise parents to medicate children with anything, including Tylenol, around time of vaccinations," Dr. Rosen said. "The further liver stress is a consideration. Over six months old, ibuprofen is OK to use, sparingly. As for fever in general, I try to help parents understand that fever is a natural way for the body to fight infection. I do not advocate the routine use of acetaminophen or ibuprofen."

- **High-pitched crying.** A persistent, inconsolable cry indicating pain that continues longer than twenty-four hours.

- **Anaphylactic reaction.** Hives, swelling of the mouth or throat, and labored breathing might be provoked by an egg allergy.

- **Rashes/Swelling.** Any red rash on the skin or large swollen bump at the injection site that lasts for several days.

- **Extreme sleepiness:** Sleeping through feedings, lethargy even when awake.

- **Vomiting/diarrhea.**

- **Behavior change.** Sudden changes in behavior or personality, tantrums, sullenness, or irritability inconsistent with past behavior.

- **Convulsions.**

- **Shock.**

- **Brain inflammation.** Blank stares, high-pitched screams, and arching of the back; often followed by seizures.

- **Physical/mental deterioration.** Difficulty performing normal activities such as talking, walking, or crawling.

After your children receive a vaccine, or series of vaccinations, carefully monitor their reactions and behavior. Keep a written record of any observations or concerns you might have—these notes might be extremely valuable later.

According to the CDC, parents "should report clinically significant adverse events even if you are unsure whether a vaccine caused the event." You can obtain information about the Vaccine Adverse Event Reporting System (VAERS) by phone (800-822-7967) or online (www. vaers.hhs.gov/vaers.htm#5). If you feel that your child might be having a life-threatening reaction to a recently administered vaccine, call 911 or take your child to the emergency room immediately.

For more information on contradictions to vaccines, see the CDC's Contraindications to Vaccines Chart (www.cdc.gov/vaccines/ recs/vac-admin/contraindications-vacc.htm). For safety information on specific vaccines, see http://aapredbook.aappublications.org/cgi/content/ extract/2006/1/1.5.18.

For more general information on vaccines, visit the National Vaccine Information Center Web site at www.nvic.org.

Vaccine Additives and Preservatives

Vaccine additives serve many different functions: they are used to stabilize the vaccine, prevent spoilage, and stop the growth of potentially harmful germs. According to vaccine manufacturers, preservatives prevent loss of potency and ensure the sterility of the vaccines. Unfortunately, far too often, many chemicals added to vaccines are also toxins that could compromise a child's health. Before giving your child any vaccine, you need to study the vaccine packaging and familiarize yourself with the various additives.

A child's reaction to various chemicals depends on several factors, including the child's age, state of health, history of exposures to certain chemicals, and heredity. If the exposure to a chemical or ingredient in the vaccine occurs at a critical time in development, even small amounts of a chemical can do great harm.

If you examine the CDC's lists of vaccine ingredients (available online at www.cdc.gov/vaccines/pubs/pinkbook/downloads/appendices/B/excipient-table-2.pdf), you'll see that some vaccines might contain some of the following ingredients, which are called adjuvants:

- **Aluminum** is used in vaccines to help stimulate the growth of antibodies that fight disease. Though it's not considered a heavy metal, like mercury and lead, high levels of aluminum exposure can cause neurological and bone damage. According to Agency for Toxic Substances and Disease Registry (ATSDR), "Children with kidney problems who were given aluminum in their medical treatments have developed bone diseases." Aluminum is also suspected of being toxic to the neurological, respiratory, reproductive, and cardiovascular systems, and has been associated with Alzheimer's disease and seizures.

The use of aluminum adjuvant in many vaccines is of increasing concern to many researchers like Dr. David Ayoub, an assistant professor at Southern Illinois University School of Medicine and medical director of the Prairie Collaborative for Immunization Safety. When combined with mercury, aluminum can produce a synergistic reaction, particularly in combination with testosterone. Dr. Ayoub has compiled a comprehensive list of the many other ways that we might be exposed to aluminum, including aluminum foil, antacids, aspirin, dust, auto exhaust, antiperspirants, treated water, vanilla powder, nasal spray, salt, commercially raised beef, tobacco smoke, bleached flour, baking powder, cans, animal feed, ceramics, commercial cheese, and of course childhood vaccines.

Dr. Ayoub also listed all of the health effects linked to excessive aluminum exposure: flatulence, headaches, dry skin, weak and aching muscles, senility, spleen pain, liver dysfunction, kidney dysfunction, neuromuscular disorders, colitis, memory loss, nervous system activity, Alzheimer's disease, Parkinson's disease, heartburn, colds, behavioral problems, constipation, numbness, and many other serious symptoms. Like thimerosal (mercury), which I will discuss in great detail later in the chapter, aluminum is likely to be the subject of heated debate in years to come, because its health effects might be as widespread.

- **Antibiotics** prevent the growth of germs in vaccine cultures, but as I explain later in the chapter, overexposure to antibiotics might lead to widespread health issues.

- **Egg protein** is used in a number of vaccines, even though some children are allergic to eggs. Because the children receive vaccines so early in their lives, their parents might not know of these allergies yet.

- **Formaldehyde,** which is also used as an embalming fluid, kills unwanted bacteria and viruses in vaccine cultures, but it is also a known human carcinogen.

- **Monosodium glutamate (MSG),** the same additive used to flavor some Asian foods, helps "stabilize" certain vaccines against heat, light, humidity, and other forces in the environment.

- **Thimerosal** (see page 135) metabolizes into one of the most toxic heavy metals in existence: mercury.

After studying this list, would you intentionally expose your child to any of these chemicals without assuring yourself that the benefits far outweighed the risks? Once you start to research these vaccine additives, you may come to the same conclusion that I have: There is still simply too much that we don't know about vaccine safety. And yet health officials keep adding more and more vaccines to the "one-size-fits-all" schedule.

Our public health agencies and the mainstream medical community in general are doing a good job of keeping watch over the "herd." You, on the other hand, are the only one who can decide what is best for your baby. So take some time to determine how vaccines and their additives might affect your child's health, particularly if you have a family history of autoimmune or neurological disorders or if you child may have a preexisting allergy to these "hidden" chemicals.

The Thimerosal/Mercury Controversy

We already know that mercury is a neurotoxin that can affect the brain, heart, and kidneys, immune system. There is also evidence to suggest that children's exposure to mercury and other heavy metals early in life might contribute to the epidemic rates of autism in this country.

Mercury exposure through vaccinations has attracted a great deal of media attention in recent years, as some parents believe that their children's autism spectrum disorders may be associated with a mercury-based vaccine preservative known as thimerosal. According to the Food & Drug Administration (FDA), thimerosal is a preservative that is 49.6% mercury by weight that's used in some vaccines to protect multi-dose vials from bacterial and fungal contamination. Until recently, thimerosal was used in three childhood vaccines: hepatitis B, *Haemophilus influenzae* B (Hib), and diphtheria-tetanus-pertussis (DTP). Hib and hepatitis B were introduced to the U.S. vaccination schedule in October 1990 and November 1991, respectively. These additions to the immunization schedule exposed many U.S. babies to mercury at levels that the Environmental Protection Agency didn't consider safe for oral consumption by adults. The American Academy of Pediatrics' *Green Book* found that "very high exposures to thimerosal-containing products have resulted in toxicity, including acrodynia [or childhood mercury poisoning], chronic mercury toxicity, renal failure, and neuropathy." When administered in a vaccine, thimerosal goes right into the bloodstream and passes through the blood-brain barrier. Once there, thimerosal—like other heavy metals—is very hard to get rid of, especially in children.

When parents found out about the health risks associated with this toxin, they became enraged, and they started putting pressure on the CDC to stop exposing children to thimerosal. In 1999, in response to these growing safety concerns, a federal program began to phase out thimerosal from most childhood vaccines, although many doses containing thimerosal lingered in the supply chain for several years afterward.

Unfortunately, the CDC's 1999 recommendation did not apply to the flu vaccine, most of which to this day contains thimerosal. And it's not as if only a small minority of children receive the flu shot. As Dr. Lawrence Rosen pointed out, it's now recommended for *all* children 6 months to five years old, regardless of their health condition.

There's a real contradiction here. On the one hand, the American Academy of Pediatrics admits that there's "no safe level" of mercury exposure; on the other hand, the CDC is recommending that we give our kids flu shots that contain mercury. But why would we *ever* inject this known neurotoxin into the bloodstreams of our children? You don't have to be a doctor to understand that the possible long-term side effects of these exposures might be extremely serious; it's just common sense. The mercury is going to do *something*. Even if you don't believe thimerosal causes autism, you must agree that injecting mercury into babies can't be good for them.

Standard vaccine policy needs to change. For the sake of our kids, we can no longer tolerate these dangerous contradictions. To date, only seven states have passed laws reducing the amount of thimerosal given to children. Until other states do the same, or until congress passes a law, we absolutely shouldn't be exposing all of these kids to this known developmental neurotoxin, especially when most of them don't even need a flu shot in the first place.

We also need to be calling more public attention to the health consequences of thimerosal. Over the last few years, scientists have begun to focus on the possible correlation between mercury exposure in early childhood and the rise of autism spectrum disorders. A recent primate study reported behavioral characteristics in infant monkeys injected with thimerosal that appear similar to autism. The Porphyrin Study found evidence of much higher than normal concentrations of heavy metals in children with autism spectrum disorders. Another significant new study by FDA scientist Dr. Jill James found that many autistic children are genetically deficient in their ability to produce glutathione, an antioxidant generated in the brain that helps remove mercury from the body.

Dr. Andrew Wakefield's research, which was published in *The Lancet* in 1998, suggests there is a possible increase in autism and other pervasive developmental disorders in children who received the trivalent measles, mumps, and rubella (MMR) vaccine. (For more studies linking mercury toxicity to autism, see p. 271 in the resources section.)

No one wants to confront these disturbing facts—not the mainstream media, not the CDC, not even most pediatricians. I keep hearing that they've "found no causal link" between mercury in vaccines and neurodevelopmental disorders. But that's a very different thing from saying that they've *proven* that thimerosal in vaccines is safe.

A year ago, I met with a prominent pediatrician and senior member of the AAP. When we started to debate this whole vaccine issue, I began by saying that, for years, children received multiple vaccinations that contained thimerosal. The total amount of thimerosal injected into the bloodstreams of these children in a single office visit far surpassed the EPA safety guidelines. How could anyone possibly reconcile that current vaccine protocol with the academy's 1999 statement that there's *no* safe level of mercury exposure? How can mercury in all forms be toxic—except when it's injected in a vaccine?

When I asked this pediatrician if anyone had ever proven the safety of these substances, he acknowledged that no one had. So then I asked him, If you don't know that thimerosal is safe, why do you continue to advocate that the Department of Health and the CDC give thimerosal flu shots?

In response, he asked me, "How will it look if we take out thimerosal from our own vaccines but continue to ship them to children in Third World countries?" Because of course our vaccine program is global, and the World Health Organization exports all of these vaccines to children all over the world.

But does this rationale make *any* sense at all? Think about the backward logic being employed here: If we're going to contaminate kids in foreign countries, then we might as well contaminate our own, too? Why can't we just stop contaminating kids altogether and devote ourselves to protecting them instead?

Until major health organizations reconsider their priorities and begin treating our children as individuals, we must remain vigilant and battle for our children's health every step of the way. In the meantime, you as a parent can take immediate action to protect your children from thimerosal and other contaminants in vaccines. Just adopt these simple rules:

Before you vaccinate, ask about thimerosal

Until thimerosal in flu vaccines is a thing of the past, you and your pediatrician have a responsibility to demand the right to a preservative-free, heavy-metal-free flu vaccine, like Flu Mist (www.flumist.com).

For Dr. Jeffrey Boscamp, the chairman of pediatrics at Hackensack University Medical Center, the issue is incredibly simple. The question of what exactly thimerosal does to children isn't even relevant, he said. "If it doesn't need to be there, then it shouldn't be there—the discussion doesn't need to go further than that. People can argue forever about whether or not thimerosal causes a problem, but still to me, it's a very simple thing—if there's any uncertainty whatsoever, and you have a choice between a preservative-free vaccine versus a vaccine with preservatives, why would you take the risk?"

Dr. Lawrence Rosen recommends the preservative-free nasal Flu-Mist, which he said works even better than the conventional flu shot.

"It's a much more effective flu vaccine than a shot," he said. "In children over the age of two years old, the injectable flu vaccine, in most studies, seems to be about 70 percent effective. Under two, it may not be more effective than placebo. There are not good studies showing that flu vaccine in kids under two are more effective than placebo."

So ask your pediatrician about FluMist, which is now approved for children as young as twenty-four months. If your child absolutely must get vaccinated for the flu, just make sure the vaccine is thimerosal-free.

Always review the vaccine packaging before immunizing your children.

Ask to see the package insert and really look at that little sheet of paper that's folded up about six times in the box. You'll find a paragraph that tells you what exactly is in the vaccine—if it contains thimerosal, or aluminum, or any other preservative. It's really easy to read. Go over this information carefully and don't hesitate to ask questions as they arise. If the vaccine contains thimerosal, or aluminum, or any other ingredient that might concern you, ask for a preservative-free alternative.

But again, don't be surprised if you meet some resistance along the way. Often, when parents demand to see this information, the nurses get offended, or they claim that they don't have the packaging, which of course isn't true.

Follow the same rule that I did: If the doctor or nurse refuses to show you the package insert, then you may want to consider looking for another pediatrician. Never forget that you are the consumer and you're buying a product from a doctor. You have the right to ask.

Get one vaccine at a time.

The system of "pooling" vaccines, or giving kids multiple vaccines in a single office visit, can overload a child's immune system, especially if that child has other health problems.

Most doctors follow the government's guidelines for vaccinations and give newborns five to seven vaccines in one visit. But in recent years, many pediatricians have begun to recommend that these vaccines be spaced out more, at wider intervals. After all, a vaccination might be perfectly safe on its own but potentially toxic when administered in combination with four or five other shots, and the combined effect of these vaccines has never been tested. Adults wouldn't accept five immunizations at once. Why would we treat our children by a lesser standard?

One of the solutions, Dr. Kenneth Bock said, is a "slower way of vaccinating—so you separate the vaccinations; get one a month, for example, rather than several of them together." Dr. Manny Alvarez agrees, saying that he advises his patients to "pace the vaccines. Don't get them pooled—avoid the three-in-one."

Until we know more about the combined effect of these powerful substances on children's already delicate, immature immune systems, you can reduce the liklihood of adverse reactions by bringing your kids in every month for the first year of their lives—it just makes more sense. After all, we're talking about babies who weigh fifteen or twenty pounds and, in the case of many preemies, whose systems are even more delicate, as little as five pounds. We need to treat these populations a little more gently. There are a whole host of health issues that just haven't been resolved.

I asked Dr. Rosen to give me an example of what he considers a safe vaccination schedule. He said that while he varies the protocol from family to family, he generally suggests the following:

- Starting at two months, one per month of pneumonococcal vaccine (Prevhar), hepatitis B, *Haemophilus influenzae* B

(Hib), and diphtheria-tetanus-pertussis (DTaP). Because each child requires three of each vaccine, separating them will take nine months. All of these vaccines will be completed by the child's first birthday.

- Second year: three for polio; three for hepatitis B (one at a time); and MMR (sometimes split, sometimes together, depending on the family's wishes) and varicella vaccine (one each).

- Check titers of all antibodies at four to five years old.

Dr. Rosen also told me that regardless of his advice, about 95 percent of his patients still opt for the standard vaccine schedule. Many medical insurers won't cover multiple office visits, and according to Dr. Rosen, there are also concerns about what's known as "standard of care." If a pediatrician actively advises a family to vaccinate on a schedule that differs from the AAP/CDC recommendations and the child contracts an infectious disease like meningitis, then the parents could sue the pediatrician, and they'd probably win. That's why parents who prefer this slower vaccine schedule might first have to sign a waiver.

But even if these precautions require a little more legwork (and doctor's visits) on your part, they are absolutely worth the extra time and effort. With our kids, it always makes sense to err on the side of safety.

Always have a long conversation with your pediatrician before giving your child any vaccine. Make sure that you understand all of the factors involved. *Don't be intimidated.*

Do not allow your doctor or his or her staff to downplay or dismiss your concerns about vaccinations. Unfortunately, some pediatricians become quite annoyed when parents question or resist some vaccinations, so be prepared to meet some resistance.

Even today, as more and more parents and health professionals are waking up to the potential hazards associated with some vaccines, there's still a lot of opposition out there. I recently asked a respected pediatrician to explain his vaccine protocol to me. Without pausing for an instant he said, "Oh, we just follow the CDC's recommended schedule."

"But what if a mother expresses concerns about thimerosal?" I wanted to know.

Again, the doctor didn't hesitate before replying: "Oh, they've taken thimerosal out of everything, I don't worry about that."

Obviously, this isn't true. There are several vaccines that still contain thimerosal including the majority of influenza vaccines; the doctor also made no mention of all the other thimerosal-contaminated vaccines he'd administered *before* the CDC recommended phasing it out in 1999.

"What if a mother expresses doubts about getting five vaccines at once? What if she prefers to have the vaccines spread out over a longer period of time?"

"Well, then," he said simply, "in that case I recommend them to another pediatrician."

But when I asked him to name the pediatrician he recommended, he couldn't—in other words, there *was* no backup pediatrician. "So you're actually turning away mothers and their babies?" I said to him. "That's it, you're simply refusing to vaccinate these children if their parents want to discuss alternatives to the standard vaccine protocol?"

His response shocked me. "Look," he said, "I don't want to be sued. I have a mortgage to pay and kids to support." In reality, the waiver that Dr. Rosen mentioned earlier—which I always signed when Wyatt was vaccinated—will protect doctors against most lawsuits, but that isn't the real issue. The real issue is that some mainstream health-care practitioners are failing to put their patients'—and our children's—welfare first.

This physician's attitude is all too common even today, when we know more about the dangers of mercury toxicity and other vaccine additives. Parents still feel too intimidated to ask legitimate questions about vaccinations. They assume that the doctors know best no matter what, that they don't have a right to demand a higher standard of treatment for their own children. But don't back down from this conversation.

For your children's sake, don't be bullied. If at any time you are uncomfortable about giving your child a vaccine or feel you are being pressured to give your child a vaccine, take a break! Tell the doctor you want to think about it.

Never forget that physicians have been wrong before. And they don't have to live with the consequences if your child suffers from an adverse reaction to a vaccine. You do . . . and more important, your child does.

As long as the medical establishment follows a one-size-fits-all vaccination policy, parents must evaluate each and every vaccine given to their children. We must do our homework and try to understand not only the vaccines themselves, and what is in them, but also the child's development, mental status, and his health status. Timing is everything, and understanding the benefits and the risks will enable you to make an informed choice about the vaccines you give your baby.

I promise all of this work will pay off in the long run. Just start asking questions about the issues that affect your children's health. Again, I'm not at all advising you against vaccinating your child. I just want you to know that in this, as in so many aspects of raising your kids, you have more options than you might think.

Spotlight On: Autism Spectrum Disorders

According to the U.S. Centers for Disease Control and Prevention, autism spectrum disorders (ASDs)—which comprise a broad spectrum of neurobiological disorders that include autisitic disorder, Asperger's syndrome, and pervasive developmental disorder (PDD)—not otherwise specified—rank among the fastest-growing developmental disabilities in the nation. As parents, we need to educate ourselves about one of the most serious health issues facing our children today.

While ASDs share essential clinical and behavioral features, they differ dramatically in severity and age of onset. ASDs, which are frequently diagnosed within the first four years of a child's life, encompass a variety of language, behavioral, physical, and neurological symptoms. These include failure to develop normal social interaction and communication, as well as restricted, repetitive, or stereotyped behaviors and interests.

Twenty years ago, autism was considered a relatively rare disorder. But recently, the number of U.S. children diagnosed with some form of ASD has risen at an astonishing rate, increasing nearly *tenfold* in the last decade alone. Every year, exponentially more kids are born with some form of ASD. Consider the following statistics:

- In 1987, the incidence of autism was estimated at 1 in 10,000 children in the United States.

- Ten years later, the rate had leaped to about 1 in 500.

- Today, an estimated 1 in 150 U.S. children has some form of ASD.

- In the first five years that the government required reporting of autism in school children ages six and above, the number of cases climbed from 5,415 to 34,101 (between the 1991–92 and 1996–97 academic years).

These figures become even more alarming when you break them up by gender: According to the National Institute of Mental Health, there are three to four times as many boys who have ASDs, which means that 1 out of every 104 boys born today will be diagnosed with some form of ASD. (A number of researchers are exploring the relationship between mercury exposure and testosterone levels, which may help account for this gender gap.) The rates also vary by region. New Jersey, for example, has the highest ASD rates in the country, with approximately 1 in 94 kids diagnosed with some form of autism.

You can't look at these numbers without wanting to ask a whole lot of questions. I know I did. What's behind these sharp increases? What causes autism and ASDs, and why do so many more kids have them than ever before?

These questions have sparked a great deal of debate—and controversy—in political and medical circles alike. What I call the "autism epidemic" has become an extremely volatile subject all over the country. No one else wants to use the word "epidemic," but when we're seeing these kinds of numbers, what other terminology makes sense?

Some organizations classify autism and ASDs as a strictly genetic disorder. But if that were true, how do you explain the dramatic rise in ASD diagnoses over the last twenty years? We've already established that there's no such thing as a "genetic epidemic"—the term doesn't even make sense. Our genes simply do not change fast enough to explain these tremendous increases.

Still others argue that there have always been this many autistic kids out there; we've just gotten better at diagnosing them. Try bringing up this point with some elementary-school teachers who've been in the profession for more than twenty years. I predict the vast majority of them will tell you that every single year, they see more and more children with ASDs in their classrooms. They'll also tell you that children with ASDs are extremely difficult to miss.

If the better-diagnosis theory were true, then where are all the thirty-year-olds with ASDs? Absolutely nothing compares to the unbelievable 1-in-150 rates that we're seeing in younger kids today. We're also seeing epidemic increases in rates of diabetes and obesity among kids today—does that all just boil down to better diagnoses as well? Were doctors just "missing" all of those children, too?

I've also heard that the recently broadened definition of "autism spectrum disorders" brings far more children under an umbrella once reserved for autistic disorder alone. "One worry," said autism researcher and director of Pieta Research Dr. Richard Lathe, "is that kids once called 'retarded' are now being called 'autistic.' But," he went on, "there's just no evidence of any diagnostic substitutions, or that our definition of autism has changed that much."

Also, look at the March of Dimes' statistics on mentally retarded children born today. Over the last twenty years, those numbers have remained fairly constant, unaffected by the out-of-control spike in autism diagnoses. If we'd just been "confusing" autism with mental retardation for all those years, wouldn't the March of Dimes' rates be dropping dramatically as more and more children were re-classified as autistic? The numbers would be in sync, and they're not.

"The other issue is awareness," Dr. Lathe went on, "and yet that doesn't fit either, because the rates get much higher as the children get younger. If you look at ten-year-olds, we have a certain rate [of children with ASDs]. If you use the same diagnostic criteria for five-year-olds, you'll see much higher rates. If you look at the number of autistic cases per year, you'll see that it steadily declines as the ages get older. Now that can't just be awareness."

"Better diagnosis is an element," Dr. Phil Landrigan told me. "You can't just dismiss it; it's there. It's part of the story, but it's not the whole story. Doctors have gotten smarter about it. But I also think there's a real increase. I think it's both. And I don't know the cause. There are lots of possibilities, but I don't think anybody truly knows the cause of the increase in autism. But the increase *is* real."

Of course doctors have gotten smarter about diagnosing autism—they haven't had much of a choice. All of a sudden, they're seeing such an incredible increase in cases of ASDs; it's only logical that they should get better at recognizing it. Whenever you have an outbreak or an epidemic of an illness, your diagnostic skills very quickly improve. That's just how it works.

A recent statistical review of fifty-four published reports of studies on autism, ASDs, and related disorders conducted between 1966 and 2003 in the United States and the United Kingdom reported that changes in diagnostic criteria or improvements in identifying cases could not fully explain the large increases in rates of autism and ASDs.

Parents' occupations might also contribute to these increases. "Historically, the parents of ASD children have tended to have odd professions—things like metalworking that increase risks of exposure," said Dr. Lathe. "It's never been fully documented, but I think there's probably a link. In the 1940s, when we first started seeing cases of autism, it was found that the parents had unusual occupations. Nowadays, I think exposure is much more widespread."

Every day, more chemicals are introduced into our environment, and we have no real understanding of how they're affecting us. Another problem Dr. Lathe mentioned is the combined effect of all these toxins together, which we haven't even begun to test. "The combination of different toxins is far more toxic than any one in isolation," he said. "So if you consider a child that's being exposed to mercury, cadmium, PCBs, phthalates—each of those might be in a safe range on its own, or well below the safe level, but all together you can get really acute toxicity."

Autism is an incredibly complex disorder, and many scientists are attributing the increase to a variety of environmental factors in combination with genetic factors or genetic predispositions, rather than any single cause. You just don't see these types of numbers over such a short period of time without *some* environmental factors coming into play.

Kids on the spectrum—all kids, really—should add omega-3 fatty acids to their diets. Cod liver oil, or fish-oil capsules, can make a big difference. Animal studies have linked diets in omega-3s to neurological problems. I recommend Nordic Naturals (www.nordicnaturals.com), whose products are free of toxins like mercury, lead, dioxins, and other heavy metals.

For more information on ASDs, visit the Autism Research Institute Web site (www.autism.com). The ARI website also has listings of DAN! (Defeat Autism Now!) practitioners nationwide.

The Rise of Childhood Allergies

Kids today have more allergies than ever before: seasonal allergies, food allergies, skin rashes, asthma, and other respiratory problems. "Allergic disorders," Dr. Lawrence Rosen said, "are increasing almost in every country in the world" at epidemic rates, especially among our children.

Allergic disorders, including asthma, allergic rhinitis, and eczema, affect more than 35 million people in this country. Every year our society spends an estimated $6 billion on treatment and another $700 million is lost in productivity at work.

But why are allergies rising at such a staggering rate? While there is definitely a genetic component to allergies, environmental pollutants also play a role. Dr. Michael Rosenbaum suggested that the almost constant exposure to multiple substances in our environment overstimulates our immune systems. "Evolution would favor a potent immune system for our ancestors, who had to fight a relatively limited set of infectious agents and allergens," he said. "That strong immune system has become maladaptive. We are exposed to high concentrations of allergens that were never there before. As a result of this overexposure to multiple environmental toxins, our immune systems have become hyperreactive even to non-toxins. What should have been sneezed out is now wheezed out. The end result is an epidemic increase in the incidence of asthma and other allergic conditions."

All sorts of triggers can cause allergies to develop. Specific environmental irritants—airborne, food, and water contaminants (including tobacco smoke, pesticides, heavy metals, pet and pest dander, food allergens) and infectious agents (viruses, molds)—along with stress interact with certain genetic predispositions to throw the immune system off balance. Allergies often result from this imbalance, and once the immune system is disordered in this way, other allergies are likely to follow.

The best approach would be to prevent this disruption from ever occurring, which you can do in a number of ways, according to Dr. Rosen:

- Limit your family's exposure to controllable allergy triggers, like tobacco smoke and cat dander.

- Use high efficiency particulate air (HEPA) filters in every room of your house to remove airborne pollutants, dust, mold spores, and other allergens from the air. A HEPA filter is especially important in the bedroom. I also recommend getting a HEPA vacuum. And make sure to replace your HEPA filters on a regular basis.

- In humid areas, use a dehumidifier to limit mold development.

- Buy allergy-proof bedding, including mattress and pillowcase covers, to reduce allergy symptoms, and regularly wash sheets, blankets, and pillowcases in hot water.

- Stuffed animals and real animals alike can contribute to allergies, so be sure to wash them frequently.

- Consider removing carpeting in bedrooms, or use area rugs that can be cleaned regularly. Vacuum all carpets and floor surfaces weekly with a HEPA-filter equipped appliance.

- Use nontoxic household cleaners.

- Eat healthy, whole organic foods with plenty of anti-inflammatory antioxidants, such as fresh fruits and vegetables.

- To prevent allergic disease in babies, consider perinatal avoidance of known food allergens, especially if there's a family history of allergies; breastfeeding might also protect newborns against allergies. Common food allergens include fish, shellfish, milk, soy, eggs, wheat, peanuts, and tree nuts like walnuts and cashews.

- Talk to your pediatrician about the use of specific natural health product supplements, like probiotics and essential fatty acids, that may lower your child's risk of developing allergies. Probiotic lactobacillus had been shown to reduce hereditary eczema and cow's milk allergies.

I also highly recommend getting a neti pot, which you can buy at Whole Foods and a number of other natural-health retailers for about fifteen dollars. Neti pots have been used for thousands of years to clean out the nasal passages without drugs. Simply combine a quarter teaspoon of noniodized salt with warm water in the neti pot and pour into one nostril. This trick will mechanically unclog stuffed nasal passages—you'll be amazed by how well it works!

I would also consider seeing an osteopath to treat allergies. Osteopathic medicine is an extremely subtle science that targets the emotional health of the whole child. A good osteopath can also help your kid deal with other issues as well: depression after the loss of a loved one, anxiety, restlessness.

Talk to your doctor about other easy steps you can take to protect your family from developing allergies.

The "Dirty Theory"

Dr. Jeffrey Boscamp, the chairman of pediatrics at Hackensack University Medical Center, proposed the "dirty theory"—also known as the "hygiene hypothesis"—as another explanation for the sharp rise in childhood allergies we've seen over the last few decades. According to this theory, children today are *too* sheltered from infectious agents in their environment. The result? Their immune systems don't have the necessary stimuli to develop properly.

"Parents," Dr. Boscamp said, "have always wanted to create a really sterile environment for their kids. The general concept was 'I'm going to put a bubble around my kids; I'm going to protect them.'"

But many recent innovations have enabled some parents to take this natural protective impulse too far. Conventional household cleaning products, like chlorine bleach, can remove too much bacteria, both the good and the bad, from children's environments. Antibacterial soaps present similar issues, according to Dr. Boscamp. "We've seen this real proliferation of antibacterial soaps—people crazed about their kids not being exposed to anything," he said. "People are now starting to think about that, too—maybe you're *supposed* to grow up around bacteria. We think of bacteria as being terrible, but in fact they're critical to our well-being. The bacteria in your intestines are *good* bacteria. They're meant to be there."

He went on: "There's this whole 'dirty theory' that you need some of those exposures—that if you take all of them away, you're going to pay a price. You're going to develop more allergies, which may mean more asthma, which may mean more sinus disease—all of these disorders snowball. I don't think that we were meant, evolution-wise, to grow up in an absolutely sterile environment. You're *supposed* to be exposed to these things as a child so that your immune system will develop appropriately." In fact, studies have shown that children raised on a farm or exposed to certain livestock may grow up to have fewer allergies than children reared in an excessively sterile environment.

I completely understand your impulse to protect your child from threats in the world around him. But remember, too much of a good thing can be dangerous.

Antibiotics Overload

Antibiotics are another potential area of concern for parents today. The invention of antibiotics represents, Dr. Boscamp told me, one of the "biggest advances of the twentieth century." Thanks to antibiotics, far fewer people fall victim to infectious diseases like pneumonia and smallpox. But in more recent years, the chronic overuse of antibiotics has become a huge problem in our culture. Pediatricians prescribe antibiotics to children for the most minor health complaints—even ones that antibiotics can do nothing to treat.

"There was always this expectation that your doctor's visit was a failed one if you didn't emerge with antibiotics," Dr. Boscamp said. But in the past five years, the situation has changed somewhat. "Parents are becoming better informed and saying, 'If it's a mild ear infection, then maybe we don't need antibiotics this time.'"

This attitude, he said, was unheard of twenty years ago. But parents and doctors alike are beginning to realize that too much of a good thing can cause problems. "Antibiotics are wonderful things," Dr. Boscamp said, "but you do pay a price for them." He went on: "Antibiotics are not dangerous to a person; the drug itself is not dangerous. There are some side effects—people can develop allergies—but that's not what bothers me. What bothers me is that indiscriminate use of antibiotics creates bacteria that are resistant to the antibiotics we use to save lives every day. Bacteria are clever: the more often they are exposed to an antibiotic, the more likely they are to change so that the antibiotic no longer works. The well-founded fear is that we will end up with bacteria that are untreatable, and we will find ourselves in the same situation we faced before antibiotics were discovered. We take it for granted that an infection can be treated, but this is not a given. When antibiotics are prescribed when they aren't needed, society pays a price: at some point, antibiotics could be useless against common infections."

Dr. Rosen agreed: "The overuse of antibiotics has created many problems, not just in pediatrics, but in medicine in general. Kids are developing resistance to many of the common antibiotics. In some cases, our first-line treatments don't work in 50, 60 percent of the kids. So then we're forced to use stronger and stronger antibiotics. The medicines themselves have a lot of side effects and adverse effects, which create other problems in the kids, sometimes worse than the infection they came in with."

And kids are just coming into excessive contact with antibiotics at the doctor's office. They are also being exposed whenever they eat nonorganic meat or drink nonorganic milk. That's why getting antibiotics out of cattle feed should become a major public-heath priority. "The idea that you're creating superbugs in livestock that will then be easily passed to humans—it's huge," Dr. Boscamp said.

He also cautioned against prescribing antibiotics to people "with an obvious viral illness—people who come in sneezing, with a runny nose, or a cold. That's really a problem because we know antibiotics don't do anything against viruses, so every time we use an antibiotic when we don't need to, we'll pay a price in the future. People are starting to understand that, to say, 'Maybe I don't need an antibiotic this time.'"

Reducing antibiotic use is one area where conventional pediatricians have come together with "green" or integrative pediatricians. Although the bias against natural therapies remains strong in our culture, more and more Western doctors have started considering alternatives to antibiotics, as well as prescribing their patients probiotics (for example, acidophilus or lactobacillus) in conjunction with antibiotics.

Spotlight On: Juvenile Rheumatoid Arthritis

Dr. Yuki Kimura, head of pediatric rheumatology at Hackensack University Medical Center, spoke to me about one of the most common (and most commonly undiagnosed) chronic childhood diseases: juvenile rheumatoid arthritis. While approximately 30 percent of the adult population of this country has some form of arthritis, people seldom realize that children might be at risk as well. Arthritis in children is an autoimmune disorder that causes inflammation of the joints.

"People are shocked," Dr. Kimura said, "that children can get arthritis. And it's even more shocking that it is one of the most common chronic diseases in children, in the top five."

There are, in fact, as many as eight different types of arthritis that can occur in children. The most common of these, oligoarticular juvenile idiopathic arthritis, most often affects little girls around the age of one or two. While oligoarticular JIA (what used to be called JRA) usually affects just a few joints, it can lead to a number of devastating complications in the eyes, including blindness.

How do you diagnose arthritis in a child? Unfortunately, detection can be very difficult. The symptom of juvenile rheumatoid arthritis, Dr. Kimura told me, is "usually pain or stiffness of one sort or another in one or more joints. Pain can be in almost any joint: in a leg, an arm, the hand joints, sometimes the spine. The problem is that kids have a hard time verbalizing their pain, especially when it begins when they're very young.

Another problem, Dr. Kimura said, is that "sometimes kids don't know that there's anything wrong, because how they feel is all they know. It's not that unusual for kids who have terrible arthritis to say, 'I don't really have pain anywhere,' because they're used to having this problem. So pediatricians and parents have to be alert about changes in behavior that might give them a clue that something like this could be going on and not wait for the child to tell them that there's something wrong. For example, sometimes a child might not express pain but they might start limping or favoring one leg over the other. Arthritis often causes stiffness after inactivity, so kids often are cranky, unwilling to walk, or appear stiff in the morning when they get up, after a nap, or after a long car ride, but an hour or two later they may seem fine." Because kids with arthritis can't always express their pain, they may not get diagnosed properly or receive the right care and treatment for it. And, Dr. Kimura said, the "earlier you treat arthritis, the better your outcome—the more likely you'll have a healthy joint for the rest of your life, as opposed to a destroyed joint."

When I asked Dr. Kimura what's behind these increases, she told me that doctors don't yet know exactly. "It's an autoimmune disease, and no one knows what causes it," she said. She added, however, that children with other chronic health problems might be more likely to develop arthritis. "I do see increases in arthritis in children who have other diseases like obesity and diabetes, or asthma, for example. But that may just be that we're seeing an increase in these diseases in the population as a whole, so I don't really see a definite connection. These are likely to be environmental triggers that we are unaware of as yet, but for now, the only kind of environmental connection with arthritis is smoking and rheumatoid arthritis in adults. Smoking has definitely been shown to be associated with increased risk for developing rheumatoid arthritis as an adult, as well as with having more severe disease."

Green Cures

As part of my effort to green my life, I have sought out alternative treatments for various physical ailments—treatments that allow me to avoid, or at least minimize, Wyatt's exposure to traditional antibiotics or other medications. Sometimes, we use these alternative treatments in conjunction with traditional medicine. I'd like to share a few of the "green cures" that I have used successfully over the years. As with all of the suggested alternative treatments in this book, I must emphasize that you should always consult your physician before proceeding to use them for the first time. A trained medical professional can guide you toward the remedies, and dosages, that might be right for your child. Every child is different, and what worked safely for our family may not be a good choice for yours.

A Green Cure for a Common Ear Infection

Dr. Rosen offered one example of a "green" treatment for one of the most common childhood complaints: the ear infection. "The conventional approach to treating an acute ear infection," he said, "is with antibiotics. When a child comes in with an ear infection, he's prescribed a potent biological antibiotic to supposedly 'kill' the bacterial ear infection. Well, there are some problems with that. Number one: Many ear infections are not bacterial. The majority may be viral or have other causes. The second problem is that antibiotics don't do a very good job of addressing pain, which is really why parents come into the office in the first place, because their child's in pain."

Dr. Rosen offered an alternative solution that spares children unnecessary exposure to antibiotics. "There are many herbal remedies that we use directly topically, on the eardrum in the ear, including garlic and mullein oil, which are safe to use and actually have been found in studies to be more effective for pain relief," he said. "Here's how I recommend parents treat an ear infection: If you can't find a reliable prepared garlic oil product to use, you can make your own. Take olive oil, put it in a pan, put a little garlic in it, crush it up, and warm it. Then, after you've let the mixture cool down, strain the garlic and put a few drops in the child's ear, using an eyedropper that you can buy in any drugstore. It works really well." Dr. Rosen emphasized the importance of letting the olive oil and garlic cool down first, to prevent burns.

When I used this extremely effective remedy with Wyatt, I had him lie on his side and covered the treated ear with cotton. After a few minutes, I removed the cotton, the ear would drain a little, and that was it.

Wyatt's ear doctor, Dr. Gwen Korovin, taught me another great technique for keeping children's ears clean and infection free: Put four drops of hydrogen peroxide in an ear dropper and have your child lie on her side with the ear that you're treating facing up. Then, put the dropper into your child's ear. In about five minutes, the peroxide will bubble up and drain out naturally. Just remember to put a towel under the ear so that the peroxide drains onto the towel and not onto your child's bed. When you're done, you can use a wash cloth to clean off the outside of the ear. That's all I ever had to do to unclog Wyatt's ears.

Curing Colic?

Dr. Rosen also provided an integrative "cure" for colic, an increasingly common problem for newborns—and their parents. "We're seeing more and more babies who have colic," he told me. "Colic is really very specific. It's not just crying, but babies who are really excessively fussy. Parents feel there's nothing they can do; they feel very helpless. Traditionally, conventionally, you treat colic by saying, 'It's OK. It'll go away in three months. Don't worry about it. Things will get better.'"

Other parents, he said, use an over-the-counter gas drops containing simethicone. Dr. Rosen does not recommend this treatment. These drops he said, can be "full of sweeteners and dyes. They're meant to dissolve gas bubbles, but research has shown that they're not any more effective for treating colic than a placebo. But yet that's the number-one thing that parents, if they're told to do something, it's that. It's usually, 'Go buy some drops, wait, it'll go away.'"

A better way to help a colicky baby, he said, is one conventional medicine often fails to address. "Look for the root causes. Why is the baby colicky? Is it just the way they're born and their temperament? No, it's an adjustment to their new environment outside of the womb. It seems to be there are some links to colic and food allergies, for example. There are links to colic and mental health issues in parents. Postpartum depression can be both linked to colic and worsened by colic. So it goes both ways.

"Moms who are depressed are more likely to have colicky babies, and colicky babies are more likely to make postpartum depression worse. We also know," he went on, "that babies who are colicky are often more comfortable if they're breastfed. But moms who are depressed are less likely to breastfeed. So it's a vicious cycle that goes back and forth."

Nutrition is one of the main topics he'll discuss with the parent of a colicky baby. "I'll ask, 'What is your baby eating?' If moms are breastfeeding and their babies are colicky, then we'll talk about avoiding certain foods, like cow's milk, or cruciferous vegetables, like broccoli or cauliflower. There's been pretty robust research showing that those babies may do better, may be less colicky and gassy and fussy. If they're formula feeding, there may be choices of formulas that are better than others."

Another approach involves herbs. "There are both homeopathic and botanical herbs that have been shown to help reduce colic in babies.

They may work through reducing stomach spasms, intestinal spasms. Chamomile's a great example. There was actually a study where they compared giving chamomile tea to babies, versus a placebo. And the babies who got the chamomile tea did much better."

Dr. Rosen also recommends infant massage, which he says is "terrific for reducing stress in babies, and in parents. It's a great way for parents to interact with the babies who may be excessively fussy." (For resources on infant massage, refer to the recommended reading section on page 253.)

Time and again, Dr. Rosen returns to the importance of a mind-body approach in addressing issues like colic. He and his patients talk about "the psychological impact that having a really, really fussy baby has on you when you're a new parent. You're already stressed out; hormone levels are flying around; there's a greater tendency toward anxiety and depression anyway. So the relationship I have with the family is very important then, because I have to talk to them. I may meet with them weekly. It's a lot about reassurance and talking about the effect that this has on a baby and a mom. So there's a real strong psychological component."

Most green doctors adopt this multipronged approach and try multiple solutions at once. "One of the differences between green or integrative medicine" and conventional medicine, he said, "is that it's not, 'Do one thing; wait two weeks; see what effect it has.' We tend to do a lot of things together. The criticism of that has been, 'Well, how do you know what works?' I'd answer that these things are meant to be used in a very holistic way, together."

When Wyatt was colicky, I found that the problem was often that he was either breastfeeding or drinking from the bottle too quickly, which let too much air into his tummy and caused discomfort. Try to slow your child down during feedings and see if there's any improvement.

If you still want to try a product, Boiron makes an all-natural colic treatment, Cocyntal (www.boironusa.com).

Essential Oil Tricks

Throughout the school year, and especially during the winter months, I use several different remedies to ward off colds and viruses. Every night before bed, and in the morning before he leaves for school, I rub the bottoms of Wyatt's feet with Thieves, a blend of essential oils by Young Living (www.youngliving.com). This precaution comes in especially handy if Wyatt is starting to feel sick or if kids in his class seem to be coming down with colds or other viruses. Follow the directions on the Thieves bottle for the recommended amount to use on your child. Like most essential oils, Thieves must be diluted when used properly, as the oils can be too harsh when used in their pure form—particularly for a child's sensitive skin. I also recommend cold-diffusing (see page 187) Thieves oil in your children's rooms for ten minutes while they are away at school. Do the same in your own room, too. Dr. Young's blend of safe, natural antibacterial oils will kill off any germs that might be lingering in your living spaces.

Because you can never be too careful during cold and flu season, I also send Wyatt off every day with a few packs of hand wipes. He uses these throughout the school day and during after-school activities. Most health-food retailers offer a selection of essential-oil-based wipes and towelettes. Unlike most leading brands of antibacterial gels and wipes, these products contain no triclosan, a disinfectant that sunlight can convert to dioxin, the most toxic substance ever tested. (An emergency-room nurse once told me that she's seen many babies come in drunk off the alcohol content in traditional toxic antibacterial products.) My family's favorite brand of natural antibacterials are Perx Organix (www.perxorganix.com), which are made from a delicious-smelling blend of chamomile, lemon, sage, and tea tree oils. We also really like the towelettes made by Herban Essentials (www.herbanessentials.com/ProductList.do).

Noni Juice

Noni, a fruit native to Tahiti and other South Sea islands, is excellent for the immune system. It contains high levels of antioxidants and helps to reduce inflammation, which is, as we know, the root cause of many serious illnesses: asthma, arthritis, even cancer. If we can reduce the inflammation enough, then we can more easily live with those diseases.

You don't have to gulp down huge quantities of noni juice to receive its benefits: one ounce a day, or even less, is usually enough to obtain noni's health benefits. You might have to get noni juice from a distributor (www.nonihealthinfo.com, www.tahitiannoni.com, and www.rawenergy .net) though it's becoming easier to find at neighborhood health food stores as well. As always, I recommend consulting a health-care professional to determine whether and how much noni is right for you. Because of noni's high potassium content, it could pose hazards to your kidney and liver, especially if consumed in excess.

The book *76 Ways to Use Noni Fruit Juice for Your Better Health* by Isa Navarre goes into detail about how much noni you should drink, and which specific medical conditions it can help treat.

A Homeopathic First-Aid Kit

Instead of masking problems with drugs, homeopathic remedies— which are very highly diluted chemically inert mixtures of everything from flowers and herbs to animal parts—strengthen the immune system and allow the body to heal itself. Homoeopaths traditionally look at the big picture: not just a person's illness, but his lifestyle, diet, and any other factors that might influence his health. The German doctor Samuel Hahnemann (1755–1843) first popularized this holistic approach to healing the body in the late eighteenth century.

Unlike most Western medicines, homeopathic treatments work over a period of time, without the instant *abracadabra* results we've come to expect from the big pharmaceutical companies. They're most effective when used as preventative measures: if, for example, everyone in your kid's class is coming down with a cold—or the flu, or even strep throat—homeopathic intervention can protect your child's immune system.

Homeopathic treatments are also safer and, in many cases, more effective than their Western counterparts. And although historically there's a strong bias against homeopathy in our culture, more and more wonderful green doctors out there are integrating its lessons—and cures—into mainstream medical practices.

With the help of several doctors who've worked with us at the Imus Ranch, I've come up with a list of accessible, affordable homeopathic products that parents can use to treat everyday childhood conditions. The majority of these homeopathic formulas are made by Boiron (www. boironusa.com), a brand that you can find at health-food stores and, increasingly, at conventional drugstores and supermarkets as well. Many online retailers carry homeopathic remedies, too, and often at discounted rates, so do a Google search to make sure you're getting the best price.

Now, obviously, I'm not playing doctor here. Yes, all of these homeopathic formulas are over the counter and low dosage by definition, but you should always consult with your physician or homoeopath before taking any new substance. Some remedies may interact with over-the-counter or prescription medicine, so make sure to tell your doctor about any substances you're taking. And the following suggestions are pretty generic homeopathy. If you or someone in your family has a particular problem, I recommend seeing a homoeopath for more customized solutions.

Please do not, under any circumstances, attempt to make your own formulations. Many herbs that are considered safe in their highly diluted, homeopathic form can be extremely dangerous in their pure forms. Belladonna, which I mention below, is a good example of this. In its pure form it is a potent poison and hallucinogenic; in its diluted, homeopathic form it gently eases pain.

I just wanted to share with you what works for my family, and for the kids who've come to the ranch. These are all great, healthier alternatives to the more familiar first-aid remedies like Neosporin and Tylenol that so many of us rely on daily.

Skin Conditions

Bruises, trauma, musculoskeletal aches and pains. Instead of Tylenol or Motrin. I use Boiron's Arnica Montana pellets. For a topical remedy, Boiron also makes Arnicare Gel, which helps bruises heal faster and soothes minor muscle aches and pains. Arnica Montana can even treat serious acute pain: One summer at the ranch, when Wyatt got bucked off a horse and broke his arm, he took only the Boiron Arnica Montana pellets for pain relief. Belladonna, an herb with many therapeutic healing properties, is another great alternative to conventional painkillers.

Bug bites and stings. Boiron's Apis Mellifica pellets help relieve minor allergic reactions and skin irritations. Boiron's Bitecare Gel is a topical treatment that I use to relieve the itchiness and discomfort caused by bites and stings.

Scrapes, burns, and minor skin irritations. Boiron's line of topical calendula remedies—which come in gel, lotion, cream, and ointment form—are really great. They can provide relief from sunburn, chapping, diaper rash, scraped knees, and excessively dry skin.

Cold sores. Boiron's Cold Sore Care Kit contains three bottles, each with a different remedy: Rhus Toxicodendron for skin and mucous membrane irritation (also good for joint pain); Apis Mellifica; and Mezereum (treats dermatitis, as well as nasal congestion).

Allergies and Colds

Allergic rhinitis or other allergic symptoms. Instead of Benadryl or other over-the-counter products filled with additives and dyes, I use Boiron's Sabadil, which works unbelievably well. I carry Sabadil tablets around with me during allergy season and just pop one whenever I feel an allergic reaction coming on.

Upper respiratory infection. Coldcalm, another Boiron formulation, is all over the place these days. For best results, I take the tablets as soon as I start to feel sick. I also like Kold Kare (www.karenherbs.com/kold_kare.htm) whenever I seem to be coming down with a cold or allergies. If your child is under the age of twelve, don't use it without first consulting your physician or homeopath. Wyatt takes Kold Kare, but only after our homeopath approved it.

Cough. A lot of pediatricians are now recommending Boiron's Chestal syrup as an alternative to heavy-duty medicines like Robitussin.

Flu. Boiron's Oscillococcinum has become a really popular over-the-counter flu treatment. Like most homeopathic remedies, Oscillococcinum works best if we head off the flu and start treating it as soon as we detect symptoms. Be proactive: I never wait until the flu has confined me to bed for a week. If I don't time it correctly, at the very moment I start to get sick, the Oscillococcinum might not work as well. If I do start taking it right away, I might still get a little cold, but I'll recover a lot more quickly.

I also use Boiron's Influenzinum during the winter. Every year, they come out with a new batch. I give it to Wyatt once a week to prevent sickness, and if he seems on the verge of coming down with something, I increase the dosage depending on my homeopath's recommendation. These remedies, combined with the essential oil protocols, usually keep Wyatt in top condition all winter long.

Sore throat or hoarseness. I use Roxalia tablets by Boiron to soothe sore throats and help relieve hoarseness.

Sinus pain, headache, sinusitis. I use Boiron's Sinusalia tablets to treat nasal congestion, sinus pain, and headaches.

Other Conditions

Nausea, vomiting, and indigestion. Boiron's Nux Vomica oral pellets work to relieve our upset stomachs.

Stress or anxiety. I find Boiron's Sedalia to be a great stress reliever. I also occasionally use the Rescue Remedy made by Bach Flower Remedies (www.bachflower.com). While I don't always like Rescue Remedy because of the alcohol content, you may wish to discuss it with your doctor. Some kids seem to do fine on it—it can even help control the symptoms of attention deficit hyperactivity disorder.

Insomnia. Boiron makes a product called Quietude. I also use Calms Forté, which is made by Hyland's (www .calmsforte.com). It works well at combating insomnia and nightmares, as well as general anxiety.

Eye irritation, dryness, or itchiness. We like Boiron's Optique eye drops as well as the homeopathic eye drops made by Similasan (www.similasanusa.com). Similasan has different products for dry eye relief, allergy eye relief, computer eye relief, and even pink eye relief. If your child has contacts, talk to your eye doctor about whether a few drops of Similasan's Dry Eye Relief will help prevent irritation and dryness.

Chapter 9

Off to School

In giving your kids an optimally green environment at home, you've also given them a huge head start on the rest of their lives. But what happens when your children go off to school and leave the universe that you've so carefully created? I believe that you can look upon this inevitable transition in two ways, as either an obstacle or an opportunity. Yes, there are plenty of hazards that you'll need to watch out for when sending your kids off to school, but there are also plenty of simple steps that you can take to minimize those hazards.

Don't let a toxic environment rob your children of what should be some of the richest years of their lives—the time when they make friends, discover new interests, grow in mind and body. As a parent, you want to ensure that your child makes the transition from home to school in the safest environment possible.

Potential School Hazards

We send our kids off to school so that they can learn and flourish in a safe, healthy environment. Unfortunately, many schools are contaminated with hazardous chemicals. Highly toxic pesticides are used on a regular basis to control pests in schools and on playing fields.

The air children breathe may be filled with the byproducts of toxic molds from water-stained ceiling tiles or carpets or poorly maintained ventilation ducts. While the common cleaning products used in schools keep the floors, desks, and hallways germ free and smelling fresh, their fumes are potentially dangerous and pose a threat to the health of our children.

Because 55 million kids in this country spend most of their waking hours in school, we need to start paying more attention to the cleanliness and safety of these buildings. The adverse health effects of toxic exposures in the schools has been well documented:

- On October 27, 1992, the Westchester County, New York, Department of Health closed down Eastchester High School for three weeks after students and staff complained of nausea, headaches, eye irritation, and respiratory problems. The day before, an exterminating company had applied the insecticides resmethrin, chlorpyrifos, and diazinon in the school.

- Asthma, which is linked to exposure to toxins in the environment, is the number-one reason for school absenteeism and the number-one chronic childhood illness.

- Conventional cleaning chemicals can contain neurotoxins, highly toxic materials that affect the nerve cells and may impair a child's developmental and learning abilities.

- A study published in the October 2003 edition of *Environmental Health Perspectives* found that teens showed a fourfold increased risk of illness from exposure to disinfectants than adults.

- Several Seattle public schools found that the lead concentration in their water fountains exceeded the 20 parts per billion recommended by the EPA.

- Many items containing mercury are found in schools. At a school in Connecticut, the simple act of cleaning out a supply closet resulted in twelve broken mercury laboratory thermometers. The school was evacuated and paid cleanup costs totaling six thousand dollars.

- A report prepared by an environmental coalition that focused mainly on five states with large school-age populations—Massachusetts, New York, New Jersey, Michigan, and California—concluded that more than six hundred thousand students were attending nearly twelve hundred public schools that are located within a half mile of federal Superfund or state-identified contaminated sites.

- Many cleaning products used in schools, such as toilet bowl cleaners, mold and mildew sprays, and antibacterial cleaners contain carcinogens, mutagens, teratogens, and neurotoxins. These substances are known to cause or aggravate cancer, cause genetic changes in cells, and affect nerve cells.

These toxic exposures can lead to school absenteeism, learning disabilities, asthma, and other chronic health problems. Remember that knowledge is your best defense against these very real threats to our children's health. Involved parents can make all the difference in bringing about the changes necessary to protect their children.

If we all join forces with other concerned parents in our

community, we can force school officials to do a better job of reducing our children's exposure to lead, mercury, pesticides, and other hazardous pollutants. There are lots of easy ways to create a safer school-day environment. Bring up your concerns with other parents at school meetings, and together you can:

- Persuade the school administration to make the switch to nontoxic and biodegradable cleaning products that contain few or no volatile organic compounds. You don't need dangerous chemicals to clean a school thoroughly and effectively.

- Test for lead in water and replace old pipes, since children tend to absorb more lead than the average adult.

- Work with your municipality to identify, collect, and recycle mercury products that might be present in your children's school. Start a drive to replace these products with nonmercury alternatives.

- Reduce the use of pesticides in school buildings and landscapes and use alternative methods of managing pests. Integrated pest management is a collaborative effort between parents, teachers, administrators, cafeteria workers, and even the students that has proven to be an effective method of managing pest infestations in school buildings, and on school grounds, without the need for pesticides.

- Make sure that the outdoor play equipment, decks, and fences at your children's schools are arsenic free. Before your child becomes ill, check the wood. You can order an inexpensive test kit to test for arsenic in the soil or in wood structures.

These tasks might sound daunting, but my environmental center can help you make cleaner, greener schools a reality. Visit our Web site (www.dienviro.com) or call us at 201-336-8071 to discuss ways to implement these protocols. We offer a free consultation and facility evaluation and can help your school green their cleaning, test for lead, switch to healthier paints and building materials, and even remake the food program.

Together, we can equip our schools to deal with these environmental threats and protect our children from harm.

The School-Day Diet

For the first few years of their lives, you can pretty much control everything your kids eat. It's not until they leave for school that most children make their first independent decisions about food. As a parent, you want to ensure that those decisions are the right ones.

Unfortunately, the typical school-cafeteria lunch—even if it has a high protein and vitamin content—is often loaded with trans fats, high fructose corn syrup, and other dangerous additives. Many schools might have chips and sodas on their menus or vending and soda machines in their hallways.

To protect your children from these toxic temptations, start by researching the foods and snacks available in their schools. If the school-day menu is for the most part comprised of processed foods, join forces with other interested parents and lobby the school's administration to make some changes—and again, my environmental center can help walk you through these essential steps. At the very least, make sure the schools are providing alternatives to junk food, and encourage the administration not to sell your children candy, soda, and fatty snacks.

Whenever you can, send your children off to school with a packed lunch. This way, you can still regulate the food that goes into your child's body when you're not around. Fresh organic produce—especially bananas, carrots, and grapes—is easy to pack and extremely portable. Sandwiches with organic, plant-based ingredients on whole-grain bread are also a hassle-free, healthy choice.

If you do send your kids off to school with a packed lunch, be mindful of the waste this can generate. According to the Green Guide, "[s]chool lunches can leave a mountain of waste, from disposable paper sacks and throwaway plastic to over half a pound of food waste per person every day." The Green Guide recommends giving your kids foods that don't require wrapping, like organic fruits and vegetables. And choose only PVC-free plastic wrappings, like the healthy cellophane wrap made from cottonwood trees sold by Green Earth Office Supply (www.greenearthofficesupply.com). And instead of brown paper bags, consider getting a few reusable (and recycled) cotton canvas lunch bags from Ecobags (www.ecobags.com). Avoid vinyl lunch boxes and bags, which may contain lead—look for the "lead safe" label if you choose a vinyl product. And instead of high-sugar boxed drinks, send your kids off to school with water in a reusable bottle. Stainless-steel bottles are safest, as reusable bottles made out of hard plastic #7 might leach bisphenol A.

But obviously, packing your kids' lunch every day isn't always possible. Food served in school cafeterias is cheap and, best of all, requires no preparation time. Since you won't be there to supervise your children's menu selection on the days when you don't have time to pack their lunches, you need to make sure that they understand the far-ranging impact of their dietary decisions early in life.

When your child is still very young, initiate an ongoing dialogue about food—I promise you these conversations will come in handy when your kids reach adolescence. Talk about why vegetables and whole grains help people function better, both in classes and in after-school activities. Practice preparing simple, delicious dishes together—make cooking a fun family activity, not a chore. Discuss the importance of drinking lots of water and avoiding fried foods.

From their earliest years, equip your kids with the information necessary to make wise dietary decisions. When you go out to dinner, avoid the items on the kids' menu, which tend to be the most toxic. Instead, focus on salads and fresh vegetables. And whether at home or in a restaurant, both you and your kids should have fresh fruit as dessert.'

As kids grow older and become more influenced by their peers, they'll be tempted by all the junk foods that are unfortunately the dietary norm in our society. So that they can resist the peer pressure they'll inevitably encounter, your kids need to know *why* they eat healthful, nourishing foods.

You should also start your child's school day off with a healthful breakfast. "It doesn't have to be elaborate," Dr. Lawrence Rosen emphasizes. He recommends including some protein to boost your kids' energy in those long hours before lunch. "School lunches and snacks should be as healthy as possible, and also include some protein, along with fresh, organic fruits and vegetables, water, and healthy whole grains if desired. Encourage your child's school to provide healthy options and avoid empty calories and unhealthy additives in most packaged snacks and beverages. Top-of-the-list things to avoid include trans fats (partially hydrogenated fats) and caffeine."

In recent years, many schools—in acknowledgement of the epidemic numbers of overweight kids in this country—have made an effort to include more healthful foods on their menus, but all too often, those options are still the exception to the rule. Or the school's "healthy alternatives" are just plain unappetizing. When kids are introduced to certain vegetables in this setting, they can develop a lifelong aversion.

"Most kids get exposed to spinach and broccoli and kale at school," Dr. Mehmet Oz, vice-chairman of surgery at Columbia University, told me. "And everything tastes bad. Beets are the best example. Beets in school taste so bad—like plastic. They're unappetizing. But you make beets with a little garlic and olive oil and a nice light cheese on it. Oh! They're just so good. But you have to make them that way, so that your kids will like them."

In other words, if you're in the habit of preparing delicious versions of these same foods at home, your kids will be capable of distinguising the good from the bad. They can dislike overcooked school-cafeteria beets and love *your* beets. So make sure your kids are getting the healthiest possible diet at home. Keep sweets to a minimum. You can just as easily satisfy your kids' sweet tooth with trail mix or fresh fruit. Remember, your children's palates develop early, even before birth. If you introduce your family to healthful, nourishing foods from the beginning, your children will be much likelier to choose those same foods on their own, even when you're not around.

For ideas on quick school-day snacks, refer to the recipes section on page 221.

Spotlight On: Childhood Obesity and Diabetes

Every year, we're seeing more overweight children in our country—a problem that will have long-term consequences throughout our society for many years to come. The last available statistics, from 2002, rank about one in six children between the ages of six and nineteen as overweight, or about 16 percent of all U.S. children. (Adult figures are even more appalling: approximately 31 percent of us are considered overweight.)

Why are we so overweight as a society? Well, for one thing, our dependence on unhealthful, processed foods has really gotten out of control. We eat fast foods loaded with synthetic preservatives and additives. Many of us—especially our kids—go weeks at a time without enjoying a nourishing home-cooked meal. We also overdo it on portion size, often eating two or even three times the necessary amount of calories at every meal. Video games and passive channel-surfing have replaced good old-fashioned sports as our national pastime.

We eat too much and move too little, and the consequences of this lifestyle are very serious and scary, especially for our kids. Overweight children are at increased risk for cardiovascular disease, high cholesterol, elevated insulin levels, and elevated blood pressure. They're also much more likely to develop chronic conditions like hypertension and type 2 diabetes as adults.

Dr. Frederica Perera described the proportion of overweight children in our society as "astonishing." Being overweight as a child, she said, "brings with it an array of metabolic illnesses—diabetes, asthma. Children who are obese at age three will likely develop asthma when they're five."

One of the most common, and most troubling, consequences of childhood obesity is diabetes, which has also risen at epidemic rates in this country over the last two decades. Diabetes is a chronic metabolic disorder that affects almost 21 million people in the United States, one to two million of whom suffer from its most severe form, called "Type 1" (also known as juvenile-onset and insulin-dependant diabetes mellitus).

One out of every fourteen people in this country has some form of diabetes, which has become the sixth leading cause of death in the United States. Diabetes can lead to kidney failure, heart disease, blindness, strokes, and limb amputations, as well as high-risk pregnancies and babies born with birth defects. The Children's Diabetes Foundation puts the cost of treating diabetes and its complications at more than $100 billion per year. And the crisis keeps getting worse. Type 1 diabetes, a genetic disease caused by a malfunctioning pancreas, used to be referred to as "juvenile diabetes."

As recently as twenty years ago, only adults had the far more common type 2 diabetes, which is much more closely linked to excess weight and improper nutrition. A child with type 2 diabetes was almost unheard of. But type 2 diabetes has increased by 33 percent in the last fifteen years. To me, that's a tragic testimony to the impact our unhealthy diets are having. A *Lancet* study published in January 2005 drew a direct link between weight gain and prediabetes and fast food menus, but somehow, we're still feeding our kids junky, high-fat foods.

Dr. Oz gave me the big picture on how excessive body fat can lead to diabetes. "The major task the body has to deal with is stress," he said. "Not just feeling stressed, but environmental stressors—toxins in our environment, foods that are toxic, emotional toxins, et cetera. A thousand years ago, the number-one stressor for the human body was famine. It wasn't deadlines or bad food; it was not having enough food. So the response that the body generates is something called the cannaboid receptors. Their nickname is the 'can't avoid' receptors. They're very powerful drivers for you to eat more, because remember, stress meant you didn't have *enough* food. You also have cannaboid receptors in the belly, in the fat inside the belly, in what's called the omentum.

"So that omentum," Dr. Oz went on, "is what makes little kids fat. That omental fat is full of these 'can't avoid' receptors. When the cannaboid receptors are stimulated there, they send back a chemical to the brain saying, 'It's OK. Calm down. We're doing fine,' which is a good thing. But they also send a chemical to the liver telling the liver to rage, to start making cholesterol, to start feeding chemicals to the body, because stress is happening. And they also block the ability of muscle to use sugar. That's called diabetes. Because it blocks insulin. So it causes insulin resistance, which is diabetes, and it causes high cholesterol levels. And those two destroy the health of kids. And we're having a lot of children with those problems now."

The diabetes epidemic is reversible, but only if we take immediate measures to improve our children's diets and exercise habits. We can save them from a lifetime of discomfort and disease by teaching them healthy lifestyle habits at the very beginning.

If your child already has type 2 diabetes and you're interested in learning about supplements to insulin injections and prescription diabetes medications, the National Center for Complementary and Alternative Medicine (a division of the National Institutes of Health) has published a report on the various natural supplements studied in the treatment of type 2 diabetes, including alpa-lipoic acid, garlic, magnesium, omega-3 fatty acids, coenzyme Q10, and chromium. You can find this illuminating report at www.nccam.nih.gov/health/diabetes.

Exercise: The Most Essential Homework of All

Along with a good diet, staying in shape is the best way to keep your kids' weight under control and protect them from the awful diseases caused by obesity. When I was growing up, physical education was a standard part of every school day. We played all sorts of sports at recess, five days a week. In recent decades, that situation has changed, much to the detriment of our kids. Across the country, when schools cut their budgets, PE is often the first thing to go. Today, very few kids play outside during the school day. Most of them spend their entire day at school seated behind a desk. Then, when they get home, they spend a few hours watching television or playing video games before settling in to do homework.

"If you go to school," Dr. Oz told me, "you'll be in gym for maybe an hour, twice a week. And of that hour, you only really exercise twenty minutes. You're not active at all. So the amount that you actually sweat is trivial. You don't have to shower afterwards, because you didn't do anything. And that's your entire activity for the week."

This situation must change. Our school years should be among the most active of our lives. Children, when left to their own devices, are in constant motion. Confining them to chairs and desks all day is unnatural, and it's also harmful. We're seeing the terrible effect this sedentary lifestyle is having on the increasing numbers of overweight kids all over the country.

So if your children's school doesn't provide them with an outlet to move around and exercise, you need to make sure they get that outlet at home.

Dr. Oz, who believes that lack of physical activity is at the root of many childhood health disorders, is vigilant about his children's exercise habits: "My daughter Zoe told me the other night that all her friends think I'm really cool," he said. "I thought there were some good reasons for this, but before I could get too flattered, she said, 'No, they think you're cool because you always tell me not to study, to come play basketball with you instead. They think it's really cool you don't ever make me study.' And I said to her, 'I don't think that—I do want you to study, but I don't want you to *only* study. I actually think physical activity is really important for you. And plus, you learn to organize yourself so that you don't have to study *all* the time for SATs or whatever you're going to be studying for in the future.'"

Dr. Oz also pointed out that children's exercise patterns are completely different from adults' patterns. "The natural tendency of a child," he said, "is not to run for an hour and then sit the rest of the day. The natural tendency of a child—the way their metabolism and bone structure and everything else is designed—is to be active all day long. They'll get up and do somersaults and wrestle for five minutes—and then they'll stop and lie around for an hour. Then they'll do the same thing over again."

Adults, he said, operate differently. "We regiment ourselves. So we took that same activity model that we have as adults, and we applied it to our kids. So we have soccer games from nine to ten, and the rest of the day, there's no activity. Whereas what a kid would normally do is play soccer for fifteen minutes and then stop. Then in two hours, they'll play again. And then they'll go and run around and chase each other, play tag—all that spontaneous stuff that we, for a lot of reasons, have taken out of our culture. And actually, the most important predictor of childhood obesity is your basic innate activity level. It's not that you're playing sports for an hour a day, but that your basic activity is higher than the other kids." He went on to give an example of this phenomenon: "If two kids were sitting in a room and the phone rang, one kid will get up, and one won't. The kid who gets up is thin. The kid who doesn't get up is not. It's that simple. That little fidgety movement is very important to the well-being of a child. And when we create an environment where that's not only not pushed for, but not enforced upon a child, then some kids won't do it." The goal, he said, should be to create the opposite sort of environment in your home—one in which constant physical activity isn't just encouraged, but required.

In past generations, schools were responsible for making sure that kids got at least some exercise every single day. Since that's no longer the case, this responsibility now falls to the parents. Dr. Rosen offers a few suggestions about how to get around this problem. "Encourage your school to think of creative ways to engage children in physical activities. Children should be involved in vigorous activities at least daily, if not several times a day. That's part of being a kid! Research has shown that physical fitness decreases the likelihood of obesity and improves attention in the classroom. Organized sports and hobbies are available everywhere and may be the greatest source of physical activity for some children; still, we must be careful to allow time for unstructured, free play as well."

Even working parents have a good range of options. If you can't be there to oversee your children's exercise, you can still find some clubs and after-school activities in your area that incorporate some form of physical activity.

And since the best parents lead by example, you can also turn physical fitness into a fun family project. I don't care how busy or overscheduled you are: Exercise is an essential part of *everyone's* life, regardless of age. As Dr. Oz points out, squeezing exercise into even the most crammed schedule provides a great lesson in time management. So start carving out a few hours a week to move around with your kids. Go on a walk through the neighborhood together, or ride your bikes for a few minutes early in the morning. Play chase in the backyard. If you live in a tall apartment building, skip the elevator and start taking the stairs once in a while. Find ways to move around more, and do it as a family.

Be creative, but whatever you do, get moving! I cannot emphasize how crucial it is that we get our kids out there exercising. As with food, our kids' relationship with exercise is formed very early in life and has a lifelong impact.

Spotlight On: Attention Deficit/Hyperactivity Disorder

Over the last few years, we've seen a tremendous surge in children diagnosed with a wide range of learning impairments and neurodevelopmental disorders. A lot of different problems fall under this umbrella, everything from mild speech delays and dyslexia to full-blown autism.

One of the most common—and most misunderstood—of these disorders, attention deficit hyperactivity disorder (ADHD), seems to be affecting exponentially more kids every year. A recent study found that almost 8 percent of U.S. children have some form of ADHD, or about 4.4 million children in all. Children with ADHD, which is often diagnosed early in the school years, often have difficulty sitting still, paying attention, and controlling their impulses. They can be overly excitable or overly aggressive. They might be restless, or talk out of turn, or have trouble completing tasks.

But despite the growing prevalence of ADHD, the condition remains greatly misunderstood. Many children might be hyperactive, impulsive, or inattentive, but within normal limits. For some, boundless energy is just a part of childhood. Other kids might have some other disorder either along with or instead of ADHD, like anxiety disorder, bipolar disorder, or even depression. (ADHD often coexists with other neurodevelopmental disorders that range in seriousness from a specific learning disability to conduct disorder.)

In recent years, some parents and medical professionals have expressed concerns that ADHD might be overdiagnosed in this country, serving as an all-purpose label for a range of different developmental and behavioral problems. Dr. Kenneth Bock, an ADHD expert, acknowledged that increased diagnosis might partially explain the rapidly-escalating rates of ADHD we're seeing. But, he was quick to add, "it's still a very real epidemic."

While doctors and researchers still don't know what exactly causes ADHD, many believe that the disorder results from a complex interaction of genetic predisposition with the environment. Nutrition might also play a big role. A study published in *The Lancet* in 2007 found that certain food additives, like the preservative sodium benzoate and colorings, can actually increase hyperactivity in children. "The finding lends strong support for the case that food additives exacerbate hyperactive behaviors (inattention, impulsivity and overactivity) at least into middle childhood," the researchers wrote. Other chemical exposures linked to ADHD include prenatal alcohol and tobacco smoke. Heavy metals might also play a role. Environmental lead and low-level exposure to manganese in areas with contaminated drinking water have also been linked to increased incidences of children with ADHD.

"I do think that toxins contribute to ADHD," Dr. Bock said. "But the difference is what we call phenotypes," or what characteristics are expressed as genes interact with the environment. "There are different phenotypes. These are different ways of manifesting physically what's happening inside. So one kid may manifest autism; one kid may manifest PDD [pervasive developmental disorder]; one kid may manifest Asperger's; another kid may manifest ADHD—all with similar contributing factors." In other words, different children exposed to the same toxins at identical levels might emerge with very different problems, or none at all.

If your child has been diagnosed with ADHD, make it your number-one priority to learn everything you can about the disorder—and what you can do to control it. Children with ADHD are often prescribed powerful medications that succeed in calming them down during school hours but might have long-term side effects that researchers are only just beginning to discover. (Source: National Institute of Mental Health)

If we clean up our children's diets, we can make a lot of progress at combating ADHD and other childhood health disorders. For dietary protocols that can help control ADHD, look into the Feingold diet (www.feingold.org, or call 800-321-3287), which John Robbins describes in great detail in *Reclaiming Our Health*. The Feingold Association of the United States is a not-for-profit organization that generates public awareness of the potential role of foods and synthetic additives in behavior, learning, and health problems. Ben Feingold, a doctor at the Kaiser Permanente Medical Center in San Francisco in the 1950s and 60s, performed many studies with children and linked 40 to 50 percent of hyperactivity to food additives. So he came up with the Feingold diet, which addresses what foods to eliminate and why. I know a mom at Wyatt's school who swears by the Feingold diet, which has helped her child a great deal. Parents of kids on the autism spectrum have also found this diet to help with gut and behavioral issues. I believe that transforming schools' food programs in accordance with Feingold's dietary principles would significantly lower hyperactivity and aggression in our kids.

The Happy Pill:
Why Are We Overmedicating Our Kids?

Instead of getting to the bottom of these problems—not just ADHD, but other issues like depression and even some autism spectrum disorders—we're prescribing powerful drugs for our children. The use of Ritalin, Prozac, and other psychotropic medications has skyrocketed tremendously over the last decade, with long-term repercussions we've yet to grasp.

These drugs certainly do help children get through the school day with a minimum of fuss. I know how it works. Say your kid is all over the place in school. He can't sit still in class; he's a constant distraction to teachers and fellow classmates; his grades are suffering. So what happens when the school principal calls you in for a conference? You're under a tremendous amount of pressure from a million different corners, you can't take time off work, and you just want the problem to go away. If you could consult one of the amazing "green" pediatricians who are sprinkled throughout our society, you might be presented with a wide range of alternatives. But unfortunately, these visionaries are still rare in the medical profession, and all too often, you're given only one option: drugs.

But giving a kid a pill and hoping the problem goes away is just a Band-Aid, not a long-term solution. I've no doubt that these drugs make day-to-day life a little easier in the short term, but they're also suppressing kids and masking the underlying causes of their problems. And very often, we know nothing about the side effects of these medications or how they'll affect kids over the long term. In many cases, they make the problem worse, not better.

Dr. Bock told me that he spends "a lot of my time trying to help kids with ADHD stay away from [Ritalin and similar medications]." He adds, however, that in some cases avoiding medication isn't possible. Still, doesn't it make sense to explore alternatives to drugs before giving them to our kids? As with so many chemicals, we haven't yet done enough research to understand what impact these medications are having.

I wish that as a culture, we'd pay more attention to the big picture. We're always looking for the quick fix, the instant-gratification answer to complex problems that require a lot more attention than we're willing to give. Conventional medicine, and of course the all-powerful pharmaceutical companies, have convinced many parents that medications, and medications alone, can prevent children from feeling depressed or misbehaving in class. Just like magic.

I've seen some scary examples of this kind of thinking at the ranch. We've had children with cancer who have also been diagnosed with bipolar disorder, or depression, or learning differences. How do doctors treat these issues? They give the kids—and we're talking about kids who've gone through chemotherapy and have already been exposed to huge concentrations of cancer medications—a prescription for Prozac, or Ritalin, or whatever else. Some kids at the ranch refer to their daily dose of Prozac as their "happy pill." A handful of them can't get out of bed in the morning without popping their Prozac first—and we're talking about kids who are twelve, thirteen, fourteen years old, kids who've survived cancer.

Every day, their behavioral patterns are the same. In the morning, right after taking their pill, they're happy, bouncing off the walls. But as the day goes on, they get more and more moody, and by nighttime, they're depressed all over again. I just can't see the positive impact of these cycles. Our kids are coming to rely on all sorts of drugs at an early age, even though we have an incomplete understanding of what exactly these drugs do. We're putting kids as young as nine years old on medications that might permanently damage their brains and bodies, just because it's easier in the here and the now.

But again, I realize that many parents see no alternative. But in so many cases, there *are* other solutions, both safer and more effective than drugs. Step back and look at the whole child—not just the behavior that's causing concern but the context of that behavior. Depression, for example, can often be the result of a hormonal imbalance, especially if a kid has had cancer, or is overweight, or has some kind of learning impairment.

The first step should be to try to find out what, if anything, that hormonal imbalance is. What's causing that deficiency? We still need to do more research on this topic, but more and more scientists believe that some kids are depressed because they haven't absorbed or metabolized enough vitamin D or essential fatty acids, so their brain doesn't function correctly, therefore their hormones don't function correctly, therefore they get depressed. Recent studies are exploring the relationship between fatty acids and mood, behavior, and personality.

Often, just a simple blood test will show if your child is deficient in a particular vitamin or mineral or amino acid or protein. Start there. If you can rule out any deficiency, then you can go to the next stage of investigating the issue.

Sometimes, the solution can be as simple as taking a dietary supplement to correct the deficiency. Because most children today live off junk foods, these deficiencies are more common than you think. Eating foods drenched in pesticides and hormones and antibiotics might also be having a damaging effect—and how will ingesting yet another chemical provide a true "cure"?

"There are a host of other potential modifiable contributors to our increasing fatness besides the increased availability of inexpensive, calorically dense foods and of devices favoring a sedentary lifestyle," Dr. Michael Rosenbaum told me. "Less sleep, the addition of artificial aromatase inhibitors and other endocrine disruptors to the environment, and increased time spent in thermoneutral environments due to heaters and air conditioners are just a few. Our bodies," he said, "are designed to maintain a delicate balance between what we eat as food and what we burn as energy, and between making a strong immune response to a serious infection but not to a dust mite. Prescription and over-the-counter medications can disturb these balances. Many psychotropic, antiseizure, antihistamine, and antidiabetic medications also promote weight gain. The steroids that someone might take to control their asthma can also increase body fat and over-suppress their immune systems, making them more susceptible to infections. Medications affect the entire body and must be used with full consideration of their possible side effects weighed against their benefits. Otherwise, they can, if not used properly, become environmental toxins."

These problems are also extremely complex and require complex responses. I'm obviously not going to tell you that in no circumstances you should give your kids these psychotropic medications—that's not what this book is about. But I am encouraging you to learn about the side effects of these drugs and to perform all possible research on alternatives to them. In many cases, you can treat neurodevelopmental disorders, as well as other issues like depression, without drugs. Talk to therapists and guidance counselors and doctors before making the decision to medicate your kid. Become more involved in your child's day-to-day life. Learn through observation what will really help him the most.

As Dr. Bock said, there's no "cookbook treatment" for the disorder. Just as there are different types of autistic disorders, there are also different types of ADHD. Some kids might be hyperactive, some inattentive, some impulsive, others a combination of all three. Treating ADHD and other behavioral problems depends very much on the individual. "You get the best results by looking at each child and trying to figure out what they need—what are their metabolic needs, their nutritional

needs, and so on. Treatment isn't one-size-fits-all—there's no one answer for every child."

Most important, since many conventional pediatricians might be
unwilling to explore alternatives to medication—which tend to be much
more time-consuming and involved—Dr. Bock recommends seeking out
an integrative doctor in your area. You can find an integrative physician
in your area on the American College for Advancement in Medicine's
Web site (www.acam.org). ACAM has a physician referral service that
covers the whole country. "Remember," Dr. Bock said, "you don't have
to settle. Find a doctor you have confidence in, who you think you can
work with."

Essential Oil Alternatives

Providing your kids with a solid foundation of proper sleep
and a whole-foods diet rich in vegetables—especially leafy
greens like kale, bok choy, and chard—is still your best
defense against the behavioral and emotional problems that
many children experience during the school years. You can
build on this foundation by introducing essential oils into
your home.

When placed in a nebulizing diffuser (which you can buy
at www.abundanthealth4u.com), essential oils can eat away
toxins in the air and actually increase the amount of oxygen in
the atmosphere. They're also wonderful at stabilizing moods
and creating a calm, relaxing atmosphere—in general, I just
find that essential oils make my home a more nurturing,
welcoming place to be. When I first walk into the house,
I immediately cold-diffuse many different oils: rosemary,
grapefruit, lavender, sage, lemongrass, frankincense, cedar,

lemon, orange, tan (a blend of clover, cinnamon, and eucalyptus). It all depends on the season or my mood at any given moment.

You can buy preblended oils, as I do from Young Living Essential Oils (www.youngliving.com), or just experiment with your own combinations. There are literally hundred of different oils that you can choose from, and as you begin to sample different ones, you'll develop your own personal preferences. Ask at your local health-food store for therapeutic-grade oils, and remember, a few drops go a long way.

Certain oils, like frankincense, can also stimulate brain cells and help improve kids' powers of concentration. At the ranch last summer, right after the last Harry Potter book came out, all the kids wanted to stay up late reading. I diffused some frankincense oil in the kids' rooms and they read for hours! Several kids liked the frankincense so much that I sent them home with a diffuser and a bottle of oil. Frankincense is a good choice for teenagers' rooms as well, especially for kids with high stress levels who spend hours every afternoon locked up in their room.

In addition to frankincense, I recommend trying some citrus oils, which are known for reducing tension and depression. (Tangerine and lemon in particular are effective at boosting moods and brightening the atmosphere of your house.) Bergamot is very relaxing and good for the nervous system, and lavender can soothe anxieties and promote sleep.

Every night before he goes to sleep, I diffuse frankincense, lavender, and lemon in my son's room. These oils help you breathe better, transporting oxygen and other nutrients into your cells and into your brain. (One major cause of disease in both plants and animals is the inability of nutrients to penetrate cells, which leads to cell deterioration, mutation, and a whole host of diseases, including cancer.) When diffused in the entryway of a house, they can destroy odors from pets, attack mildew, and absorb airborne dust particles. It's the healthiest, cleanest way to deodorize your home.

You can also refresh your kids' sheets and linens with essential oils diluted in water. Add six to eight drops of your favorite essential oil to a small (6- or 8-ounce) spray bottle, fill with water, shake well, and squirt as needed. Again, there are countless oils to choose from. A lot of women like rose, which is a more expensive oil; for kids' rooms, grapefruit is a really popular choice. For more ideas, refer to my favorite book on essential oils, Dr. Young's *Essential Oils Desk Reference*.

Treating Head Lice

Roughly 6 to 12 million people in the United States are diagnosed with head lice each year, mostly children aged three to twelve years. Head lice don't cause disease, though the persistent itching can lead to bacterial scalp infections. But the lice themselves are not dangerous—just uncomfortable and annoying.

So why are we treating these essentially harmless pests with incredibly concentrated toxins? The most common agents used to treat head lice, pyrethroids, are synthetic insecticides that can cause dizziness, nausea, and headaches. Dr. Phil Landrigan told me that the two leading brands of head-lice treatments contain the "very nasty chemical" hexachlorobenzene. We're talking about agricultural pesticides here—the very last substance we should be rubbing into our children's scalps!

Why would we *ever* expose our children to such powerful toxins? Probably because head lice still carry a persistent stigma in society. Parents are under a great deal of pressure to get their kids "nit free" in three days, or else the kids aren't allowed back in school. But we're paying too high a price for this convenience.

More and more people are beginning to rethink our traditional head-lice treatment protocol. Several states are considering bans on lindane, the organochlorine pesticide in one popular lice-treatment product, as a suspected carcinogen and neurotoxin that bioaccumulates in the environment and might cause seizures and deaths in humans exposed to it. But we still have a long way to go. Malathion, another main active ingredient in conventional head-lice products (and also flea-control products for pets), is an organophosphate insecticide that might be toxic to the endocrine, neurological, gastrointestinal, and respiratory systems. Malathion also breaks down into an even more dangerous compound, malaxon.

Until the mainstream medical community unanimously recognizes the dangers that these chemicals pose to school-age children, we need to protect our kids from them ourselves. My environmental center is working hard to get the efficacy of a natural product recognized by doctors. With the help of Dr. Jeffrey Boscamp, our resident head-lice expert, we're conducting a large-scale research project to test the product—a healthy alternative to traditional treatments containing toxic pesticides such as lindane and malathion—in schools. In the beginning stages of the project, we'll be surveying parents at several New York City schools, as well as approximately 2,700 school nurses in New York and New Jersey, about their experiences treating and diagnosing head lice. Then, in certain schools, we'll begin a trial study with a natural head-lice treatment that has worked well in clinical tests in Israel. If we succeed in proving that this nontoxic treatment is as effective as the toxic alternatives, we hope to get this natural treatment listed in the American Academy of Pediatrics' Red Book, so that physicians can recommend it.

In the meantime, focus on prevention first. Don't wait until your kid gets lice to deal with the consequences. The shampoos that Wyatt uses all year round contain essential oils that naturally repel lice, so that even when a lice infestation is going around his class, he always comes home lice free. Avalon Organics (www.avalonorganics.com) makes wonderful shampoos and conditioners that smell great and help repel lice naturally. The rosemary, lemon, and ylang-ylang formulas are incredibly effective at repelling lice. You should use these shampoos all year long, but particularly at the beginning of the school year and following winter break, when lice outbreaks most often occur.

If despite these preventative measures your child still comes home with lice, you shouldn't ever in any circumstance resort to toxins. Here's what Dr. Lawrence Rosen recommends you do: "Mix any or all of the essential oils of tea tree, ylang-ylang, anise, rosemary, marjoram, sage, and eucaplyptus—all of which have demonstrated anti-lice properties—in a coconut oil base. You can add a little lavender if you'd like, to improve the scent. Mix with a small amount of shampoo and apply as a rinse to the child's head. Leave on for 15–30 minutes, then wash out. Repeat daily for one week."

In addition to using this nontoxic mixture, I also recommend wet-combing through your child's hair thoroughly. Get a fine-toothed comb and run it through your child's hair regularly for the duration of the infestation, several times a day to remove eggs. You can also look into battery-operated lice combs. Just stay away from the toxins.

I only went to the hospital once in my whole life. When I was in second grade, I came home with lice. My mom went out and bought an anti-lice shampoo, and when I was rinsing it out of my hair, a little bit got in my eye. I started shrieking and screaming at the burning sensation, and even after I finally stumbled out of the shower, I couldn't see out of my left eye. When my mother saw my eye, she drove me straight to the emergency room. The doctors saw me right away and cleaned out my eye, but I didn't regain my full eyesight for another week. At least I got to wear a pirate eye-patch over my left eye for the rest of the month!

—Geoff K., San Francisco, CA

Pesticides on Playing Fields

To keep those playing fields where our kids participate in sports and other activities looking so green and trim, maintenance workers regularly spray them with a cocktail of synthetic poisons: fungicides, herbicides, and insecticides. In fact, every year, this country produces more than *1 billion* pounds of pesticides, which makes these concentrated agricultural chemicals—which can be toxic to fish, wildlife, and humans—extremely hard to avoid.

Still, we can, and must, fight to protect our kids from unnecessary pesticide exposures, since according to the American Academy of Pediatrics' Green Book, "[E]pidemiologic studies have found associations between certain cancers (e.g., brain cancers, non-Hodgkin lymphoma, and leukemia) and pesticide exposure."

And if you think your children are somehow escaping exposure to these chemicals, think again. The Centers for Disease Control found residues of numerous pesticides in the bodies of 15 percent of the children tested. What's worse: the broken-down products of these organophosphate pesticides showed up in a jaw-dropping 98.7 percent of the kids tested. Do we really want our children coming into contact with these powerful toxins? I certainly don't.

Before taking action against these harmful practices, you should first familiarize yourself with the pesticide laws in your area. Mostly thanks to concerned parents across the country, more than four hundred school districts have now implemented policies mandating integrated pest management, a toxin-free pest-control method, or an organic lawn-maintenance policy. If your school district doesn't fall into this category, contact the watchdog organization Beyond Pesticides (www .beyondpesticides.org) about changing that. Join with other parents and petition your local schools about doing a better job of protecting your children.

Spotlight On: Asthma

With air pollution, both indoors and out, so out of control in this country, rates of asthma have also increased sharply in recent years, particularly among the most susceptible population, our children. According to *The New York Times*, the prevalence of childhood asthma rose from 3.6 percent to 5.8 percent of children between 1974 and 1997—more than a 60 percent increase. Around the world, the overall prevalence of asthma rose 100 percent between 1985 and 2001.

Now a major public health problem, asthma affects nearly one in thirteen school-age kids, making it the most common chronic childhood illness in the United States. It's the number-one cause of missed school, responsible for 14.7 million missed school days every year. In Canada and the United States, five children die from asthma every week.

Like many of the diseases affecting our children today, asthma is caused by a combination of genetic and environmental factors. Allergens, viruses, preexisting food allergies, and poor air quality can all trigger asthma in a susceptible child. Because their exposure to these irritants tends to be greater, low-income populations, minorities, and children living in inner cities have disproportionately high rates of asthma and disproportionately higher morbidity and mortality rates associated with asthma as well.

"Different ethnic and economic groups are more affected by asthma than others," Dr. Frederica Perera told me. "In 2001, the prevalence rate of childhood asthma was around 8 percent in the country as a whole. In Harlem, 25 percent of children were asthmatic. Asthma rates tend to be higher in lower socioeconomic groups." Access to care is one reason for this discrepancy, she said, but "there is also the issue of disproportionate exposure to pollutants that can cause and later trigger asthma." African-American children between the ages of five and fourteen are nearly four times likelier to die of asthma.

Asthma is like most allergies, much easier to prevent than to cure. To reduce your child's vulnerability, work to eliminate all potential asthma triggers in your home, like cockroach dust, mold, pollen, cat dander, certain foods (milk, eggs, soy), and tobacco smoke. Dust mites and microscopic insects that lurk in bedding and furniture also contribute to the asthma epidemic in this country.

On the other hand, homes that are *too* clean might also put a child at risk for asthma. Remember the "dirty theory" or "hygiene hypothesis" I discussed in the previous chapter? Well, it applies to asthma, too. Lay off the heavy-duty chemical cleaners and antibacterial products. To develop properly, a child's immune system does require some exposure to bacteria.

These prevention tactics are all the more important because, once your child has asthma, she's more likely to develop not just other allergies, but a range of different health problems as well. "Everything is interlinked," Dr. Manny Alvarez told me. "An asthmatic kid can't go to school, can't exercise and play with his friends in the backyard, so he's not burning calories. So what does he do? He opens up a bottle of soda, and he eats, and he watches cartoons." That couch-potato kid is more likely to become overweight, therefore more likely to come down with all the adulthood health problems that result from obesity.

If you do suspect that your child might be asthmatic—and almost 80 percent of childhood asthma cases are diagnosed before the age of five—take her to see her pediatrician right away. Have a long talk with your doctor about how to recognize and control the symptoms of asthma, and make sure that you pass on this information to your child and other family members. If left unchecked, asthma can wreak havoc on every aspect of a child's life. It can interfere with schoolwork, extracurricular activities, and of course sleep.

So talk to your pediatrician about a plan for managing asthma, and then stick to that plan. Together, you and your child can learn to recognize common asthma-attack triggers, like excessive stress or emotion, cigarette smoke, cold air and other climate changes, respiratory infections, and exercise.

Green School Gear
Environmentally Friendly School Supplies

Especially as they get older, you want your kids to be aware of the choice you've made to green their lives. One way to do this is to purchase eco-friendly school supplies. The fantastic Web site www.ecomall.com has lots of suggestions for taking your consumer eco-consciousness into the classroom. It lists good eco-friendly school supplies, like recycled paper made without chlorine bleach; reusable pens; binders and notebooks with cardboard covers; nontoxic markers; and white glue. It also has school supplies to avoid, like epoxy glues, chemical dyes, and plastic notebooks and binders. You can find good ecological school supplies at an increasing number of stores and Internet vendors:

Office Depot (www.officedepot.com) has a good selection of eco-friendly school supplies, including Foray Recycled Groundwood Construction Paper and recycled multipurpose printer paper.

Office Max (www.officemax.com) also has recycled postconsumer-waste printer paper. Whenever you buy paper, always look for the recycled-content and chlorine-free symbols.

Green Earth Office Supply (www.greenearthoffice supply.com) is a really fun source for eco-friendly supplies. You can find hemp notebooks, paper-making kits, recycled lined notebook paper, refillable mechanical pencils, and even pencils made from recycled jeans and recycled lunch-trays. Green Earth Office Supply also sells recycled rubber portfolios, binders made from recycled cardboard, circuit-board, pressboard, and a bunch of other cool items your kids will love.

GreenLine Paper Company (www.greenlinepaper .com) also has a great selection of green office supplies, from 90 percent postconsumer-waste recycled pencils and recycled plastic pens to a variety of tablets and notebooks made out of paper.

Clothing and Accessories

The next time you hit the stores for back-to-school clothes, think about buying your kids a few wardrobe basics made out of organic cotton. Yes, it's more expensive, but cotton is the most heavily sprayed crop in the country, so for certain items, like jeans and T-shirts, you really should investigate some organic options, since the pesticides often linger in the fabrics even after many washings. If you shop online, try Lapsaky (www.lapsaky.com) for an extensive selection of organic baby and children's clothing. Earthpak (www.earthpak.com) makes backpacks, computer bags, and duffel bags from recycled plastic bottles, and Eco Goods (www.ecogoods.com) has a few nice organic cotton and hemp socks, sandals, and jeans.

Textbook Swaps

At the end of the year, start a textbook recycling program for the books your kids won't use again. We spend an insane amount on required-reading texts for schools and very often dispose of those books at the end of the school year, while younger kids are going out and buying the exact same books! It's a huge waste of resources and money. Start a swap in your neighborhood and see how much you'll save!

For bigger-scale conservation efforts, encourage your children's schools to get involved in the wonderful Green School Project (www .greenschoolproject.com), which pays schools and other organizations for their used printer, fax, and copier cartridges, cell phones, and other electronic equipment that would otherwise build up in landfills. If you can convince your school's administration that the Green School Project will save money, you might find some very willing listeners. This program could serve as a great fund-raising tool.

Greening Your After-School Activities

You can also educate the next generation about the urgent necessity of taking better care of our earth by starting an after-school club. Internationally renowned eco-activist Jane Goodall has had incredible success with her Roots and Shoots (www.rootsandshoots.org) club, which has chapters in more than one hundred countries. Roots and

Shoots' motto, "The power of youth is global," says it all for me. If we can just get our kids motivated about environmental issues, we can make a huge difference in the future of our planet. Roots and Shoots organizes hands-on educational activities for school-age children interested in environmental issues.

The National Wildlife Federation has another fun program, Backyard Habitats (www.nwf.org/backyard/), which teaches kids (and their parents) how to tranform their backyard into a veritable wildlife refuge. These and other ideas could all deepen your kids' dedication to a greener environment. As they get older and more independent, your kids should learn to engage in environmental issues on their own terms.

Chapter 10

Adolescence and Beyond

Help! You've done everything right, and suddenly your child has become unrecognizable—almost a complete stranger. But please, don't panic. It happens to the best of parents. Your precious baby is just going through a little thing we call adolescence.

I started this book with an emphasis on getting back to the basics, and at no point is this philosophy more essential than when your children hit adolescence. You want to make sure that, by this pivotal stage, your teenagers respect their bodies, have a healthy relationship with food and exercise, and maintain open channels of communication with you. In his book *Understanding the Messages of Your Body: How to Interpret Physical and Emotional Signals to Achieve Optimal Health*, Jean-Pierre Barral expresses one of my core beliefs about raising and educating our children: "Just as we teach our children respect, politeness, various rules of civility, and other ways to get by in school and in society, we have to teach them the right attitudes to promote their well-being and health." Barral goes on to sums up these "right attitudes" brilliantly, in just a few well-chosen words: "eat healthily, sleep well, breathe deeply, move harmoniously." Those are the basics for you right there.

Of course, even if you embrace these principles and hope for the best, the teenage years still won't be easy. They never are. If your teenagers never once yell at you, or slam the door in your face, then they just aren't doing their job. What you need to focus on is *your* job, which is to always be there for your child, no matter what. Now that your kids are finally growing up and preparing to make their own way in the world, they shouldn't just view you as a disciplinarian. They should also see you as a teacher, a counselor, and a friend. Peer pressure can be a tremendously powerful force during the teenage years; you need to make sure that you still have some influence, too.

Remember Barral's lesson: "Parents who know how to explain and give good advice don't need to forbid." Try to keep this simple truth in mind throughout your child's adolescence. Make it your goal to dispense advice, not prohibitions; love, not judgments.

Diet and Lifestyle

Throughout this book, I've discussed the importance of healthy eating and exercise habits. For me, it all comes back to the basic lifestyle choices we make and the values we impart to our children. Nowhere is the impact of these decisions more evident than during the teenage years.

Kids who eat well are less likely to develop eating disorders or become overweight. These days, so many teenagers, especially teenage girls, are obsessed with having the "perfect body"—an impossible image dictated by the magazines that they read and the television shows they watch. In pursuit of this perfection, they obsessively count calories while subsisting on diet cola and toxic snack foods. Even scarier: they also might develop a dependency on natural-health supplements for weight control or bodybuilding. The use of these unregulated substances, which increases every year, can lead to cardiac problems. These "natural" supplements might also be contaminated with lead or steroids.

Don't let these practices be an option in your household. A healthy diet can do wonders for your child's self-esteem and help prevent these problems. It can also help stabilize moods and minimize the hormonal disruptions that can lead to some of the scariest trends among teenagers today, like severe depression and self-destructive behaviors like "cutting" (slicing the skin with razor blades or box cutters) and "huffing" (inhaling the propellants from aerosol cans). A healthy, balanced lifestyle is the key to ensuring that our kids feel good about themselves and their bodies.

I wasn't raised a vegetarian, but my mother never, ever let me or my brother touch fast food—she lectured us nonstop about how awful and unhealthy it was and made sure that none of our friends' parents gave it to us. When I turned sixteen, I felt like the last kid in America who had never once gone inside a McDonald's or Burger King. So what was the very first thing I did when I got my driver's license? That's right, I pulled up to the drive-thru of the nearest fast-food restaurant and ordered a huge, greasy bacon cheeseburger. "If only my mom could see me now!" I thought gleefully. I parked my car and ripped right into the bag of delicious-smelling food. Unfortunately, the fun stopped there. The hamburger was disgusting—I couldn't believe this is what my friends had been eating all those years! After about three bites, I threw the whole bag away, and I felt sick to my stomach for the rest of the night. I've never told my mom about this illicit trip to the drive-thru window, and I probably never will. I still don't know if I should be grateful or resentful that she spoiled my taste for fast food forever!

Mary B., Silver Lake, CA

The Power of Fitness

No matter what their level of athletic ability, all teenagers should participate in a sport or some other regular physical activity. I'm not saying that your child has to be an Olympic athlete—far from it. But if your kids are out there exercising every day, feeling good and comfortable in their bodies, they're far less likely to abuse substances when they become teenagers. If you exercise regularly, you just respect your body more—it really is that simple.

Kids in good physical condition have higher self-esteem, and kids with high self-esteem are less likely to engage in sexually promiscuous behavior. Kids who stick to a regular regimen of exercise also do a better job of managing their time. And because they have more energy, physically fit kids are also less vulnerable to depression than kids who spend twenty-four hours a day slumped over a desk or vegetating on the couch.

If your child doesn't like team sports, explore other options in your neighborhood. There are tons of different activities worth trying for kids who have outgrown the parks and Little League teams. Martial arts, yoga, biking, even belly dancing—be creative about finding your kids an appealing activity that, with any luck, they can enjoy for the rest of their lives.

Whatever you do, make an effort to fight the couch-potato complex that's so pervasive in our culture. High-school students seem to spend the majority of their waking hours surgically attached to computers, cell phones, MP3 players—so much so that they don't notice what's going on in the world around them. Getting your teenagers involved in a sport or any other athletic activity is an effective means of combating our increasingly sedentary ways, all the while fostering a sense of belonging and achievement.

Stress and Self-Reliance

Instilling a strong work ethic at an early age is the most important gift you can give your child. No matter what financial resources your children start out with in life, they need to learn to work hard. I don't know what my life would be like if my parents hadn't instilled that work ethic in me: I had a paper route for most of my childhood, from fourth grade through high school. Every single day of the year, my brother, sister, and I were all responsible for different household chores. And during high-school summers, I always had a job. And sure, I complained a little at the time, but today, I think that work ethic and sense of discipline is the single most valuable lesson my parents ever taught me. By the time I reached high school, I could easily manage my schoolwork with sports and my paper route—I'd been juggling multiple commitments for years by then.

Sometimes, I worry that we're raising kids today to be passive participants in the world—teaching them to be entitled, spoiled, and lazy. It's too easy to go soft on them, to excuse them from any real responsibilities. But in the end, you're actually hurting your kids by not making them work for their place in the world. Responsibility is empowering, and a solid sense of accomplishment is absolutely crucial in building a child's self-esteem.

At the ranch, we teach kids the value of discipline, structure, and self-reliance. And it might seem surprising, but most kids actually *like* the lessons of discipline we instill. At first, they grumble a little, like I did when my parents first assigned me chores, but by the second day, they're jumping out of bed at 5:30 a.m., eager to go muck out the stables. Kids benefit from structure—they don't like sitting around in a chair all day. Hard work teaches them how to be engaged and enthusiastic.

These lessons become even more important when kids reach high school, because an ability to work hard is instrumental in helping kids manage stress. The vast majority of doctors I interviewed commented on the sky-high stress levels of kids today. "Children today are under more stress than at any other point in history," wrote Dr. Lawrence Rosen. "They have more schoolwork and activities scheduled than ever before, [and a] lack of unstructured free play, especially in natural spaces, adds cumulatively to these factors. Stress contributes directly to adverse health effects, including numerous pain (headaches, abdominal pain) and mind-body syndromes (anxiety, depression, ADHD, eating disorders, suicide, and homicide)."

Dr. Rosen is absolutely right. The world we live in—and are raising our kids in—is more stressful than ever before. Kids are given more schoolwork and expected to participate in more extracurricular activities than at any point in our history. Media overstimulation can seriously hamper our children's mind-body development: with iPods, video games, and televisions running twenty-four hours a day, many of them never get a chance just to sit back and collect their thoughts, much less go outside and sweat. On top of that, they're expected to have perfect grades, get into the perfect college, and have their whole existence figured out by the age of eighteen.

These competing, impossible pressures—and nonstop distractions—are taking a major toll on our children, nurse Barbara McGoey told me. "Children are under a lot of the same stress that we had as kids, but it's put on them earlier. They're in daycare earlier; they're not with their parents as long; they're in after-school programs. You have to do well in sports; you have to do well in school. You have to, have to, have to. I mean, you have a baby now and people are like, 'What? You don't have them registered for the perfect preschool by the time he's two?' And I just want to say: Stop. Why can't he stay home and watch *Sesame Street* with mommy? There's nothing wrong with not having your child in preschool. But we're just pushing society at such a helter-skelter rate, and sometimes the kids just can't handle it."

By the time our kids reach adolescence, these unrealistic expectations can boil over, sometimes with dire consequences. "We're just seeing more and more kids depressed, more and more kids trying drugs to escape," McGoey told me.

Dr. Rosen believes that rest is just as important as any scheduled activity, particularly when the new school year gets under way. To avoid getting overwhelmed by all their responsibilities, kids need time to unwind and destress. Kids today, he said, "are so overscheduled—some towns even have had to set aside one day a year for families to stay home after school and relax."

A more practical solution, he said, is "to incorporate some regular, routine way for children to destress during each and every day. It doesn't have to be another scheduled activity, though yoga classes are popular, but simply a quick and easy method for relaxation. I teach many of my patients an easy, five-minute breathing exercise they can practice at home. Turn off the TV, unplug the video games, and enjoy some quiet time; that's my prescription for a well-balanced start to the school year."

By the time your kids are in junior high, these relaxation techniques—just like the work ethic—should be long established in your household, because the pace of your kids' lives isn't going to slow down as they get older. On the contrary: Every year, their lives will only get more complicated and stressful.

As a parent, you want to teach kids how to manage all the demands placed upon them. As always, the best way to do this is to lead by example. No matter how busy (or stressful!) your life seems, you or your partner should always make time for a sit-down dinner with your kids. Show them that stress doesn't always have to equal shutdown. This nightly ritual not only reinforces your kids' healthy relationship with food, it also allows you to touch base regularly, which is crucial during the teenage years. The whole meal can last a total of twenty minutes, but those twenty minutes can make all the difference in the well-being of your child.

A lot of the problems teenagers face, from substance abuse to sexual promiscuity, can be curbed with early intervention. Just by carving out a little bit of time every day, you can prevent many of these problems from ever taking hold.

Spotlight On: Precocious Puberty

Every year, our children are growing up a little faster—not just psychologically, but physically. Premature sexual development has become a fact of life in recent years, especially for African-American children. "In one human generation," said Sandra Steingraber, "we have dropped the age of breast development by one year and a half."

Increasingly, according to *The New York Times*, "some physicians worry that children are at higher risk of early puberty as a result of the increasing prevalence of certain drugs, cosmetics and environmental contaminants, called 'endocrine disruptors,' that can cause breast growth, pubic hair development and other symptoms of puberty." Devra Davis told me that "pediatric endocrinologists have actually proposed defining breast growth in a six-year-old black girl and a seven-year-old white girl as normal. Because it's become so common—breast growth that you would get in a thirteen-year-old on a six- or seven-year-old is now considered normal.

"We have to understand," she went on, "if something's causing breasts to grow on a baby girl at age one or two, then it's stimulating breast growth inappropriately."

Researchers have much more to learn about what exactly is causing this premature puberty. Skin creams and shampoos containing hormones have been isolated as particular culprits, but as the phenomenon becomes more and more widespread, scientists are beginning to exam-

ine higher-volume exposures as well, like chemicals used in manufacturing processes.

But we absolutely must learn more about this troubling trend, because premature sexual development is not without grave health risks.
According to a report Steingraber prepared for the Breast Cancer Fund,
girls who reached puberty early in life might be 50 percent more likely
to develop breast cancer later in life.

Until we definitively understand the root cause of precocious
puberty, we must, as always, try to protect our kids from dangerous
chemical exposures. Keep your kids away from chemical personal-care
products and make sure they're eating right and getting enough exercise.

Toxic Temptations

As your kids grow more independent and drift into the "real world,"
they'll face a lot of the same dilemmas that you did years earlier. Help
them make the most of their new autonomy.

Personal Care Products

If you've taught your teenagers how to make consumer decisions with
foresight and care, they should already have the savvy to examine labels
before bringing any new personal-care products into the home. But
unfortunately, with all the societal pressure to look perfect around the
clock, some teenagers—especially teenage girls—begin to buy products
indiscriminately. They'll snap up any potion that promises to make
them prettier, and by extension more popular, no matter how toxic.
Eight-year-old girls are dyeing their hair and getting manicures on a
regular basis. And boys aren't immune to Madison Avenue's influence,
either. Last summer at the ranch, I was shocked by how many of them

were spraying themselves in completely toxic, foul-smelling "body sprays." Just five years ago, I'd never even heard of such a product.

Nail polish, mascaras, perfumes, hair dyes, moisturizers, foundations—all of these popular personal-care products might contain any number of dangerous toxins, including diethanolamine (DEA), a suspected carcinogen; formaldehyde, a known carcinogen; neurotoxic heavy metals like lead and mercury; and various types of parabens, a preservative that can act like estrogen.

Like many girls her age, seventeen-year-old Jessica Assaf estimates that she was using around thirty products every single day by the time she was twelve. When she learned how little the government was doing to regulate the cosmetics and beauty products she depended on, Jessica took action, banding with other concerned students in her Northern California community to start the organization Teens for Safe Cosmetics (www.teens4sc.org). Among other impressive feats, Teens for Safe Cosmetics was instrumental in the passage of California's Safe Cosmetics Act, which was signed into law in October 2005.

Jessica is a real inspiration to me. Her story proves that passionate teenagers can make a concrete difference in shaping the future of our planet. So get your kids engaged in the issues affecting our world today. Encourage them to develop their own opinions and stand up for what they believe in.

Vaccines

Even as your kids become independent, you still need to take an interest in issues that affect their health and safety. You should pay attention to new vaccines like Gardasil, which the FDA approved in 2006. Gardasil protects against the four types of human papillomavirus (HPV), which causes 70 percent of cervical cancers and 90 percent of genital warts. The problem is that we don't yet know enough about the

HPV vaccine's side effects or the additives it contains. Don't get me wrong, I'm all for cancer prevention. But several states have tried to mandate the HPV vaccine for teenage girls, and I don't believe that vaccines should ever be mandated. Whether your child is fifteen months or fifteen years old, you should always have a long discussion with your doctor about the benefits, and risks, of any vaccine. Only then can you decide what's right for your child.

Substance Abuse

Experimentation is a completely normal part of childhood. But in recent years, teenagers have started abusing a record number of substances: cigarettes, alcohol, illegal and prescription drugs. Some teenagers abuse substances to help them cope with sadness or the impossible stress of their lives, or to compensate for low self-esteem. Some do it to keep their weight down, or to get attention, or to appear more mature. Whatever their initial motivations, teenagers can suffer for many years as a result of these destructive behaviors.

Kids are naturally curious about trying new things, and they're also extremely susceptible to peer pressure. But by adolescence, your child should be able to tell the difference between substances and activities that heal the body and those that do damage. If, as I mention earlier, your kids are eating right and getting out there and exercising every single day, they're far less likely to start smoking cigarettes (like 3 million other teenagers in this country!) or abusing alcohol or drugs.

Keep an eye on your kids. Talk to them about these issues whenever you can, and always without preaching. Nurture their self-esteem so they don't feel the need to venture down these dangerous paths. Remind them that they have their whole future in front of them.

Indoor Environment

Teenagers are prone to locking themselves inside their rooms for hours and hours on end—it's just a fact of life. To ensure that their bedroom is as safe and healthy as possible, clean regularly with nontoxic substances. Don't let the junk and dust pile up in their private lairs. Teach them about the benefits of diffusing essential oils and keeping their belongings neat and orderly

Future Preparations

As your teenagers grow older, you'll inevitably have to start making preparations for the time when they leave your house to start their own lives. Whether their next step is college or a job, you need to supply your teenagers with the right tools for a safe, healthy future.

One way to do this is to go shopping together. At the beginning of this book, I wrote that the consumer has supreme power in this society. By controlling what we buy and what we bring into our houses, we are making a difference in the world around us. So if we buy organic meals and nontoxic household cleaners, we're raising the demand for these products and helping to lower the price of them, too. If you haven't already, make a point of teaching your teenager about these principles whenever you go shopping for food, beauty products, or even clothing.

Another idea, to promote the healthy-eating angle, is to institute a few at-home cooking lessons for your family. Get everyone involved. Teach your teenagers how to prepare the foods they love for themselves. Then, when they go off into the world on their own, they won't fall into the bad habits that have so many college freshmen gaining ten pounds. (Dr. Oz's daughter, Daphne, wrote a great book, *The Dorm-Room Diet*, about how to beat this trend.) Wyatt can already make some of his favorite meals without any help from us. We supervise him, of course, but he does all the cooking on his own.

And whatever you do, keep the dialogue open with your kids. Maybe they know more about environmental issues than *you* do. Talk, and don't forget to listen.

Chapter 11

Beyond the Home:
Community Activism and Outreach

Taking charge of your household environment is the essential first step in any greening process. If you teach your kids good eating and lifestyle habits, they'll have a fantastic head start in life. Unfortunately, individual action isn't always enough.

That's why it's important for parents to "take control in a broader sense" of their children's environment. Together, we can work to change attitudes and promote healthier living on a larger scale. "Engaged parents can really move and shake policymakers," said Dr. Frederica Perera.

There are lots of easy ways you can work to bring about changes in your community, and the benefits are enormous. You can organize petitions for organic food, or lobby your local government for cleaner buses. In fighting for these changes, you'll also be acting as a role model for your kids and teaching them invaluable lessons about the importance of taking responsibility for the world they live in.

Advocate for Organic Foods

Visit your local health-food store to find a wide range of organic, environmentally safe products that are free of toxins and other threats to your child's well-being. Search your neighborhood for organic food stores and farmer's markets to purchase your produce and meats. If you find a farmer's market that suits your needs, be sure to ask them if their merchandise is organic, since some farmers use pesticides and other toxins.

But if there isn't a health-food store or organic market in your community, you can take steps to remedy the situation. Submit a petition signed by parents to local grocers, requesting that they designate a section for organic products. It's really that easy—if more people understood how effective petitioning can be, they'd no longer accept food contaminated with toxic fertilizers and other chemicals.

This grassroots movement is how the whole organic-foods movement got started in this country. Concerned parents banded together and demanded organic foods, and soon enough, the stores began stocking them. I promise you, this approach works. It's a basic principle of capitalism: If stores think their customers will buy a product, then they will stock it. It's really that simple. Never forget that it's the consumers, not the manufacturers, who are ultimately in the driver's seat.

Campaign for Cleaner Air

"Many parents have become involved in clean air community campaigns," Dr. Perera told me. "They've lobbied to get trucks to stop idling in front of schools and lobbied for cleaner buses. Some of our partners here have used our data on the effects of airborne pollution on the developing fetus and young child to change policies in neighborhoods and in New York City, getting cleaner buses. You see our cleaner-energy buses looking proud on the streets." Why not launch a clean air campaign in your area, too?

Carpool

Whenever possible, organize carpools to take your kids to school and other activities. Take public transportation whenever you can, or carpool with colleagues to work. Carpooling helps reduce your family's carbon footprint, and it also builds community, saves time, and lowers stress. Taking the high occupancy vehicle lane will bypass traffic and shorten your commute.

Green the Cleaning at Your Children's Schools

Teachers and administrators have your children's best interests at heart and will be responsive to your concerns. Parents who've lobbied their children's schools to replace toxic cleaning products with environmentally friendly alternatives have a great track record of success. If enough concerned parents speak up, school administrators will listen. Again, for advice on how to do this, contact my environmental center (www.dienviro.com).

Begin a Recycling Program

Many households waste resources—a society-wide problem that has a significant cumulative effect on our environment. To reduce your household's waste, turn recycling into a fun activity that the whole family can take part in. Subdivide your trash into glass, plastic, aluminum, and paper and teach your children why recycling is important. Most communities routinely pick up these recyclable materials. Inform other parents of the days and times these pickups occur and encourage them to begin a recycling program in their homes as well.

If your neighborhood doesn't have regular recycling pickups, find a recycling center near you and take recyclable products there yourself. Or, even better, lobby your local government to improve its recycling policies. Make sure your office and schools have adequate recycling programs in place as well. And if you have a backyard, consider starting a compost pile for organic kitchen waste.

> *Educating ourselves and our children on the importance of recycling/reusing is a difficult job in such a disposable country. Giving old toys/clothing away to charities or even having garage sales is a good start. When shopping for items for the family, teach them that buying a used item is giving it new life and a new home!*
>
> *Julie S., Dallas, GA*

Advocate for Green Urban Development

Just as you and other concerned parents in your community can make organic foods more widely available in your area, you can also advocate for more tree plantings, parks, and sidewalks in your community. Get involved with urban development in your neighborhood—I promise you it will make a difference. There are higher incidences of obesity in neighborhoods without sidewalks and parks, since kids with no access to public outdoor space often don't have the opportunity to move around as much. There's a lot you can do to make your neighborhood healthier for the next generation. Start circulating petitions. Attend city-council meetings, and talk to your local lawmakers. Everyone benefits from greener neighborhoods.

Start a Local Community Garden or Farmer's Market

People are always talking about the importance of buying locally grown fruits and vegetables, and I agree that local food is far healthier than food that has been transported in planes and trucks and been stripped of many of its nutrients in the process. Unfortunately, in many communities buying locally just isn't a realistic option yet. In small towns all over the country, people just don't have access to farmer's markets. And even if they do, the items on sale—soaps, flowers, baked goods—can be both expensive and nonessential.

You can get around this problem by starting a garden or farmer's market in your community. That's what people did in Santa Fe, and it's been a huge success. A project like this can really bring the whole community together. You can swap talents and recipes, trade ideas and products. You might be surprised by all the different skills people have and all the creative energy this sort of undertaking can generate. For more information on starting a local farmer's market, see http://edis .ifas.ufl.edu/fy639 and www.organic-growers.com/start_a_farmers_ market_l.htm.

Support Child-Friendly Legislation

Our government can help us in our fight to protect our children. In the resources section, I go into detail about many laws—from the Conquer Childhood Cancer Act to mercury-free vaccine legislation—geared at preventing childhood illnesses. I cannot emphasize how important it is for you to support this legislation, both on the state and federal levels. Write your congressional representative and senator so that they understand that children's health should be a priority—not just for parents, but for everyone.

Whatever steps you take to green the world around you, remember that it's not just about the here and the now. It's about leaving a cleaner world for your children, and theirs, to inherit. Greening your baby is the best decision you'll ever make.

three:
resources

Food

Stocking Your Kitchen

There's no time like the present to start cooking healthier! I always prefer cooking at home for quality control and purity. You never know what goes into the food served at restaurants. Preparing your own food is a great way to ensure that your family is getting a healthy, well-balanced diet.

It's good to stock your home with a variety of delicious—and nutritious—staples. For items that don't need refrigeration, I recommend you buy a few dozen glass Ball jars, which you can find at most houseware stores. Ball jars come in sizes ranging from four to thirty-two ounces and usually cost about a dollar each. Keep a dozen of these jars filled with healthy snacks out on the counter, or in the panty, so that your children can have easy access to their contents. Fill each jar separately with your favorite nuts, seeds, and dried fruits, and as always, make sure everything's organic.

Nuts and Seeds

- Sunflower seeds
- Raw almonds

- Tamari almonds

- Raw filberts

- Raw cashews

- Raw walnuts

- Raw pecans

- Raw pumpkin seeds (or lightly baked with olive oil and salt)

- Ground flaxseeds (we sprinkle flaxseeds on absolutely everything)

Dried Fruits (buy in bags or from the bulk bin)

- Dates

- Dried pineapple

- Dried banana chips

- Dried cherries

- Dried blueberries

- Fresh fruit. Keep a variety of in-season fruits in a bowl on the counter so that everyone has access to it.

In the Fridge

- Fresh fruit. That's right, even more of it. You can never have enough!

- Organic eggs. Buy farm-fresh, local eggs from free-range hens that have been out of a cage all day and have been fed only organic vegetarian feed. A good brand to try is Wild Oats organic cage-free eggs (www.wildoats.com).

Natural Sweeteners

Stay away from foods high in artificial sweeteners and high fructose corn syrup. Your family will all love these healthy alternatives.

- Agave nectar
- Stevia
- Maple syrup, Grade B
- Evaporated cane juice
- Lundberg's Sweet Dreams brown rice syrup (www.lundberg.com)
- AH!Laska organic chocolate syrup (www.ahlaska.com)

Flours

I like to keep a variety of flours on hand for baking. Try these healthier alternatives to bleached white flour:

- Spelt
- Oat
- Whole wheat
- Unbleached

Grains

Whole grains are an essential part of a healthy plant-based diet. Refined grains, by contrast, are among the worst processed foods, adding calories and quickly digested sugars without much nutritional value. You should also keep these in glass jars in the pantry—they all make great foundations for easy, affordable meals. And again, buy exclusively organic ingredients whenever you can.

- Barley
- Bulgur
- Brown rice
- Rice pasta
- Jasmine rice
- Whole wheat pasta
- Soba noodles
- Quinoa
- Millet
- Wild rice

Beans

Many stores sell beans in bulk. Look for the big plastic bins in the bulk-food aisle. Beans are a delicious—and inexpensive—staple of a healthy, plant-based diet.

- Black-eyed peas
- Green lentils
- Red lentils
- Black beans
- Kidney beans
- Pinto beans
- Navy beans

- Split peas
- Popcorn

Other Proteins
- Tofu
- Tempeh

Organic Nondairy Milks
- Unsweetened Silk Soymilk (www.silksoymilk.com)
- Strawberry Banana Vitasoy soymilk (www.vitasoy-usa.com)
- Edensoy Carob Soymilk (www.edenfoods.com)

Extras for Cooking
- Annie's Organic yellow mustard (www.annies.com)
- Annie's Organic horseradish mustard
- Apple cider vinegar
- Bionaturae organic extra virgin olive oil (www.bionaturae .com)
- Bionaturae tomato paste
- Bionaturae crushed tomatoes
- Bionaturae strained tomatoes
- Eden Organic sauerkraut
- Creamy and whipped Earth Balance butter (www .earthbalance.net)
- Herbs: Fresh or dried organic nonirradiated herbs, especially

basil, clove, fennel, garlic, parsley, turmeric. (At our house, we put turmeric—which has antiinflammatory and anti-cancer properties—in everything from tofu and scrambled eggs to soups, pastas, and potatoes.)

- Imus Ranch chips and salsa (www.imusranchfoods.com)
- Imus Ranch balsamic vinaigrette
- Mediterrean Organic wild capers (www.mediterreanorganic .com)
- Muir Glen organic ketchup (www.muirglen.com)
- Muir Glen fire-roasted tomatoes
- Natural Value Dijon mustard (www.naturalvalue.com)
- Organic tamari
- Spectrum Organics mayonnaise (www.spectrumorganics .com)
- Spectrum Organics canola oil
- Spectrum Organics safflower oil

Beverages and Juices

The average American gets one-fifth of his total daily calories from beverages. Most popular beverages—sodas, juices, shakes, and even coffee drinks—are packed with sugars or artificial sweeteners, artificial colors, and other additives. I avoid these beverages and stick with good old-fashioned water, which is calorie, sugar, and additive free. If you want flavor, try adding a slice of lemon or lime or some fresh-cut herbs (mint is delicious). If you do drink juice, look for 100 percent organic fruit juice that has retained its pulp (that's where most of the nutrients are found) and is additive free. You can cut calories and reduce tartness by mixing it with water. Here are some of my family's favorite drinks:

- Lakewood organic pineapple juice (www.lakewoodjuices.com); Bionaturae organic nectars (strawberry, Sicilian lemon, and wildberry, at www.bionaturae.com); R. W. Knudsen Just Black Cherry juice and R. W. Knudsen Very Veggie low sodium organic juice (www.knudsenjuices.com)

- An assortment of herbal teas, both in bags and in bulk. Watermelon and chamomile teas are excellent for babies, toddlers, and children of all ages. Since he was about a year old, Wyatt had loved watermelon tea with a little agave nectar stirred into it. He loves to drink the chamomile at night before bed, or whenever he feels restless and wants to relax.

- Imus Ranch coffee

- School-day drinks: Instead of sending your kid to school with a disposable box of juice, give them plain filtered water in a reusable container. Those cardboard boxes create a ton of waste, and the juices themselves are loaded with sugar (even if it's natural). If you still prefer the convenience of juice boxes, some of my favorite brands are Whole Kids organic juices (www.wholekids.com.au/organicjuice), Edensoy soymilk boxes (www.edenfoods.com), and Silk soymilk boxes (www.silksoymilk.com).

Fresh vegetables

Fresh veggies should be a staple of your whole family's diet. As soon as you decide to have kids, make a particular effort to start eating more leafy greens like kale, Swiss chard, and bok choy.

- Beets
- Bok choy

- Broccoli

- Daikon

- Carrots

- Cauliflower

- Celery

- Collard greens

- Dandelion

- Jalapeños

- Kale

- Onions

- Peppers (red, yellow, and orange)

- Potatoes (Yukon gold, fingerlings, Idaho)

- Scallions

- Spinach

- Sweet potatoes (Jewel, Japanese)

- Swiss chard

Recipes

Breakfast Ideas

Healthy Breakfasts on the Go. The following ideas are all breakfasts that you can realistically prepare even on the busiest mornings before school. Wyatt loves every single one of these meals. And always bear in mind that you're not just passing on tastes to your kids: You're also passing along behaviors. Your kids' relationship with food is formed by how you eat. If you eat in a rush standing up, then your child will do the same. If you skip meals, then so will your child. If you always have seconds, your child will, too. So no matter how crazed your weekday mornings might become, make a point of sitting down to eat breakfast with your children. Turn the most important (and usually most rushed) meal of the day into an opportunity to model healthy eating habits.

- **Mochi**, or Japanese brown rice puffs, are a great breakfast staple. Mochi bake-and-serve rice squares are dairy free, wheat free, and gluten free and have no cholesterol. They come in different flavors like raisin cinnamon, plain, and chocolate. To prepare, all you do is pop them in the oven and bake for eight to ten minutes. You can find mochi on the web (www.grainaissance.com/mochi.html) or in health-food stores.

- **Oatmeal.** You can buy organic ready-cut oats in bulk for just a few dollars. To prepare, cook oats in boiling water for three minutes. Turn off the heat, then add a tablespoon of agave nectar, a teaspoon of ground flax, put in cereal bowl, and serve. You can top with fresh organic berries if you'd like.

- **Smoothies.** Smoothies are ideal breakfasts and after-school snacks. Even in the winter, your whole family can enjoy the benefits of an energy- and antioxidant-packed smoothie. In your blender, combine a cup of organic soymilk, a broken-up banana, organic frozen berries (Cascadian Farm is a great choice), a tablespoon of flax oil or ground flax, and a little plain organic soy yogurt. You and the kids can drink the smoothies right before walking out the door—it's a great way to start your day.

- **Ezekiel live grain bread.** Spread some organic almond butter or jam over the slice for a delicious morning treat.

- **Cantaloupe and strawberries.** Cut up and serve in a cereal bowl.

- **Berries and yogurt:** Combine a cup of berries with some organic plain yogurt in a cereal bowl. Add a little ground flax and agave, then mix everything together with a spoon before serving.

- **Organic grapes and mochi:** To add sweetness, pour some agave nectar on top of the little mochi puffs and organic grapes.

- **Organic hot chocolate:** Heat up organic soymilk for two minutes, add Ah!laska hot chocolate mix or several squares of organic dark chocolate and serve it to your child in the same mug every time. You can pair the hot chocolate with organic enchiladas or some other yummy leftover.

Basic Biscuits

Our chef at the Imus Ranch, Arlena Teitelbaum, makes delicious homemade biscuits. For more on Arlene's recipes visit www.NourishSantaFe .com).

Preparation time: *10 minutes*

1 cup organic unbleached flour

1 cup organic whole grain flour (buckwheat, oat, spelt)

2 teaspoons aluminum-free baking powder

½ teaspoon sea salt

6 tablespoons organic coconut oil

¾ cup organic nutmilk or soymilk

Preheat oven to 400°F. Sift dry ingredients together. Incorporate solid oil into crumbled mixture. Add liquid to dry mixture and stir loosely. Do not overmix. Drop onto greased baking sheets and bake 10 to 12 minutes.

Bountiful Biscuits

Follow the same instructions as Basic Biscuits. Add any variety of dried fruits, nuts, or seeds.

Balancing Breakfast Bars

These bars take a little longer to prepare, but they freeze well, and kids love them. Another great Arlena Teitelbaum recipe.

Preparation time: 25 to 30 minutes

2 ripe organic bananas

2 tablespoons organic cinnamon powder

1 teaspoon sea salt

1 cup organic agave nectar

1⅓ cups organic flaxseed, finely ground (flax meal)

⅓ cup purified water

1 cup organic sweet potato or pumpkin, mashed

2 cups organic carrots, shredded

2 organic apples, peeled and finely diced (or shredded)

3 cups organic rolled oats

1 cup organic oat flour

1 cup organic spelt flour

1½ cups organic almond butter

¾ cup organic coconut flakes

¾ cup organic walnuts (or pecans), finely chopped

Preheat oven to 350°F. Combine bananas, cinnamon, salt, ¾ cup agave nectar, 1 cup flaxseed, and water until smooth. Add the sweet potato, carrots, and apples. Add oats and flours until fully incorporated. Grease a glass lasagna pan and bread pan. Place mixture into pans and spread/pat until evenly distributed (about ½" thick). Bake for 50 to 60 minutes. While the bars are baking, prepare the icing. Mix together the almond butter, remaining agave and flaxseed until smooth. Cover and set aside. When bars are cool spread almond mixture on top and then sprinkle with coconut and nuts. Cut into small rectangles to serve.

Granolas

Granolas are great for breakfast or for a snack any time of the day. Mix and match ingredients and see what your child likes best. Store-bought granolas can have a high fat and sugar content, and it's a cinch to make your own at home. Some possible ingredients:

- Organic walnuts or pistachios and dried cherries
- Organic almonds (raw plain almonds mixed with tamari almonds)
- Organic pumpkin seeds
- Organic goji berries with raw pistachios (I call this one "Christmas granola")
- Organic dried pineapple chunks
- Organic banana chips

- Organic dry rolled oats mixed with walnuts, almonds, raisins, dried pineapples, blueberries, or cherries

- Organic dried mango and filberts

Rio Grande Granola

For a more elaborate granola, try the one we make at the ranch. The kids all love its slightly chewy texture, fragrant spicy taste, and perfect amount of sweetness. Before baking, the mixture is somewhat sticky, so use a big wooden spoon to stir it. Store in an airtight container until you're ready to enjoy it.

Preparation time: 15 minutes
Cooking time: 30 to 35 minutes

2 cups rolled oats

¼ cup raw unrefined sugar

¼ cup raisins

¼ cup toasted almonds

¼ cup sliced dehydrated banana (optional)

1 tablespoon ground cinnamon

⅛ teaspoon ground ginger

¼ cup safflower oil

1 to 2 tablespoons honey

½ teaspoon vanilla extract

Preheat the oven to 300°F. Combine the oats, sugar, raisins, almonds, banana, cinnamon, and ginger in a large mixing bowl; stir until blended. In a separate bowl, stir together the oil, honey, and vanilla. Add the wet mixture to the dry mixture and stir with a wooden spoon until well blended. Then spread the mixture in a thin even layer on a large baking sheet and bake 30 to 35 minutes, until lightly browned, stirring it twice and then patting down with a spatula. Scrape the granola onto a clean baking sheet and set aside to cool. Makes six ½-cup servings.

Healthier Snacking

If you're careful about the nutritional content of your children's diet at mealtimes but let them eat any old junk for snacks, you're not developing their palates properly. Kids should eat nourishing foods *all* the time, not just at the dinner table.

Store-Bought Snacks. Fresh whole foods are always preferable, but unfortunately not always a realistic option. The good news is, quite a few companies make some very healthful, nourishing snacks. These are some of my favorites:

- **Oskri Organics** (www.oskri.com) makes wonderful sesame-seed bars in a variety of flavors: molasses, date syrup and cumin, date syrup and fennel, molasses and fennel, molasses and black cumin, and fennel. Your child can start snacking on these bars, which contain brown rice and are very high in iron, from the age of four or five. Oskri makes lots of other naturally sweetened snacks that make great alternatives to the toxic candy bars most kids eat every day.

- NuGo (www.nugonutrition.com) makes organic nutrition bars in lots of great flavors: orange smoothie, banana chocolate, and peanut butter, in addition to the basic vanilla and chocolate.

- **Carob Edensoy Milk** (www.edensoy.com).

- **Edward and Sons** (www.edwardandsons.com) makes great organic brown rice snaps and other wholesome vegetarian snacks. The brown rice snaps comes in flavors like vegetable, cheddar, toasted onion, salsa, and black sesame.

- **Mary's Gone Crackers** (www.marysgonecrackers.com) crackers with caraway seeds are excellent.

- **Late July** (www.latejuly.com) also has great organic crackers in classic rich or classic saltine flavors. Try the crackers with organic almond butter and an organic kosher dill pickle for an extra treat.

- **New Morning** makes honey grahams with organic grains and no hydrogenated oils. For a great school-day snack, put two full graham crackers and some organic tamari almonds in a brown waxed-paper baggie. You can find New Morning products at www.mannaharvest.net.

  School-Day Snacks. You can mix and match the following organic ingredients according to your child's preference. Put them in Natural Value unbleached wax paper baggies, which you can buy at most health-food stores and on the web at www.naturalvalue.com/Pages/Nonfoods.html, www.amazonnatural grocers.com, or, www.organickingdom.com. These portable foods all make great alternatives to the junk foods most schools consider acceptable snacks:

- Dried figs (mission and Calimyrna)

- Dried dates

- Dried strawberries

- Chunks of celery, carrots, and apples

- Olives (black, red, green) tossed with chunks of tofu or soy cheese and Edward and Sons brown rice snaps

- Granola is great for packing into your child's lunch box for a wholesome treat at school. Just put some in a waxed-paper baggie, fold over the top, and send your kid off to school with a truly nourishing treat. Try any of the granola combinations listed in the previous section, or experiment and invent your own!

Mr. Martin's Maple-Glazed Pecans

Use these crunchy sweet pecans on salads, with desserts, or on stir-fried veggies. You can use the same recipe to make glazed walnuts, as well. This is a popular recipe at the ranch.

Preparation time: 3 minutes

2 cups raw pecans

½ cup maple syrup

¼ cup raw unrefined sugar

1 tablespoon salt

Preheat the oven to 350°F. Spread the pecans on a baking sheet and toast until lightly browned and fragrant, 8 to 10 minutes. Remove them from the oven and set aside. Heat the maple syrup and sugar in a medium saucepan over medium heat, stirring frequently, until boiling. Boil the mixture for 2 minutes, and then add the toasted pecans. Continue cooking, stirring to coat the pecans, about 30 seconds more. Spread the pecans onto a baking sheet to cool. Sprinkle with salt. Makes about 2½ cups.

Imus Ranch Guacamole

This guacamole is super easy to make. To prevent darkening, squeeze some fresh lemon juice over the top of the guacamole before covering and refrigerating.

Preparation time: 8 minutes

4 ripe avocados, peeled and pitted; combine Hass avocados and fuerta avocado (lighter-skinned avocado)

3 tablespoons fresh lemon or lime juice

4 cloves garlic, minced

1 tablespoon chopped cilantro

salt, to taste

Combine the avocados, juice, and garlic in a medium bowl; mash with the back of a fork or potato masher. Add cilantro (optional), and salt, and mix well to blend flavors. Cover and transfer to refrigerator. Serve cold. Makes 4 cups.

After-School Snacks. Here are a few ideas for snacks and light meals that you can prepare at home in under fifteen minutes:

- **Soy yogurt and granola.** For at-home snacks, mix plain soy yogurt with raisins, cashews, ground flaxseeds, or any of the other ingredients you use in your favorite granolas. You can also mix in some rolled dry oats for added texture and fiber.

- **Smoothies:** We love smoothies at my house, and not just for breakfast. We combine organic frozen berries with soymilk, agave, ground flaxseed, and a banana. The results are always delicious.

- **Tofu "cheese" salad:** Cut up organic tofu mozzarella-style, in chunks, and combine with fresh tomatoes and Greek olives.

- **Pita breadsticks:** Cut spelt-bread pita into strips, brush them with olive oil, then sprinkle salt, pepper, and soy parmesan on top. Bake in the oven for 10 minutes or until crispy and crunchy.

- **Yellow rice:** Cook jasmine rice with lots of turmeric powder for a natural antioxidant meal.

- Sheets of Kombu or Nori organic seaweed

At the ranch, Arlena makes sweet, healthful snacks that all of the kids (and cowboys) love. Here are a few of the perennial favorites.

Arlena's Nourishing Truffles

Preparation time: 10 minutes, plus 15 minutes to roll truffles
Refrigeration time: 1 hour

1 cup organic shredded coconut

3 tablespoons local bee pollen (or toasted almonds, coarsely ground)

8 tablespoons organic carob and/or cocoa powder

⅓ cup hot water

10 tablespoons organic almond butter

5 tablespoons organic brown rice syrup

3 tablespoons organic vanilla extract

2 tablespoons organic agave nectar

Combine ⅔ cup coconut and bee pollen (or almonds). Set aside. In a mixing bowl, combine carob and/or cocoa powder with hot water. Stir until completely dissolved. Add remaining ingredients. Mix thoroughly. Refrigerate mixture for an hour. Roll into 1-inch balls and set on tray lined with unbleached waxed paper. Dip each ball into coconut mixture. Store finished truffles in the refrigerator and enjoy up to 7 days.

Arlena's Caramel Popcorn

Preparation time: 12 minutes

3 tablespoons organic sunflower or canola oil

¾ cup organic popcorn (unpopped)

½ teaspoon sea salt

6 tablespoons melted Earth Balance natural spread

3 tablespoons organic evaporated cane juice

2 tablespoons organic blackstrap molasses

¼ cup organic agave nectar

Preheat oven to 225° F. Heat sunflower oil and popcorn on medium high in a large stainless-steel pot with a tight-fitting lid. Move the pan around so the popcorn is coated with oil. Allow the corn kernels to begin popping. As they start to pop, turn the heat to medium and move the pan back and forth over the burner until all the kernels have popped. Next, pour popcorn into a large stainless-steel or glass bowl and sprinkle with sea salt. Melt Earth Balance in pan and whisk in remaining ingredients. Pour mixture over popcorn, stirring the popcorn until it is evenly coated. Place coated popcorn evenly on two baking sheets lined with unbleached parchment paper. Bake on middle oven rack for 15 minutes. Allow to cool and then transfer to glass containers.

Simple Smoothie

Preparation time: 5 minutes

1 ripe organic banana

¾ cup unsweetened organic soymilk

⅓ cup organic orange juice

Using a food processor or blender, pulse the banana until chopped. Add soymilk and pulse until mixture starts becoming smooth. Add orange juice and pulse until frothy. Serve immediately. Note: "Pulse" is a feature on many blenders, but simply turning a food processor on and off will produce similar results. Overblending the bananas creates a heavier, thicker smoothie.

Blue Moon Treats

Every child (and adult) should be entitled to a little self-indulgence every once in a while—what in my house we call "blue moon treats." Rather than deny your child his favorite treat, save these indulgences for special occasions, enjoying them only once in a blue moon. Here are a few of my family's blue moon treats:

Root Beer Float. We love Virgil's Root Beer, which is a great alternative to junky sodas. Virgil's is a blend of spices, anise, licorice, vanilla, cinnamon, clove, wintergreen, sweet birch, molasses, nutmeg, pimento berry oil, balsam oil, and oil of cassia. The only sweetener used are the molasses (which has lots of iron) and the natural sweetness of the birch and vanilla. Virgil's is gluten free, too.

To make the root beer float, put two scoops of vanilla Soy Delicious ice cream in a parfait glass or tall drinking glass, then pour the Virgil's root beer all over the ice cream and serve with a straw. This blue moon treat is as simple as it gets but oh so satisfying.

Walnut Chocolate Chip Cookies

Preparation time: 12 minutes
Cooking time: 10 to 12 minutes

1½ cups unbleached white flour

¾ teaspoon baking powder

½ teaspoon salt

¾ cup trans-fats-free margarine

¾ cup unrefined white sugar

1½ teaspoons vanilla extract

1 egg

1 cup rolled oats

¾ cup chocolate chips

¾ cup chopped walnuts

Preheat oven to 375°F. Sift together the flour, baking powder, and salt. In the bowl of an electric mixer, combine the margarine, sugar, and vanilla.

Beat on medium for 2 minutes, or until creamy. Add the egg and continue beating until the mixture is glossy, about 1 minute. Stir the flour mixture into the margarine mixture until well blended. Then stir in the oats, chocolate chips, and walnuts. Drop the batter by rounded tablespoons onto a cookie sheet 2 inches apart. Flatten the cookies with floured fingers and bake 10 to 12 minutes, or until golden. Remove from the pan and cool on a rack. Makes 2½ dozen.

Hot Fudge Sundaes. I make these with organic soy ice cream, AH!Laska's organic chocolate syrup (www.ahlaska.com), and soy whipped cream. Choose your favorite cut-up fruit for toppings: coconut, kiwi, strawberries, bananas, raspberries, whatever you prefer.

Sunspire Organic Chocolates. I used to eat M&Ms for my blue moon treat, but now I've gotten healthier even in my indulgences. These days, I reach for Sunspire's dark-chocolate-covered blueberries and dark-chocolate-covered almonds (www.sunspire.com).

Organic Potato Chips. There are lots of great lines of organic chips out there. I love the sea salt and vinegar chips made by Kettle (www.kettlefoods.com).

Fried Veggies. This is one of our absolute favorite blue-moon treats—frying sliced leeks, zucchini, eggplant, and tomatoes in a homemade batter. We use either organic breadcrumbs or we make our own breadcrumbs out of leftover organic bread. Mix the breadcrumbs with an egg and add sea salt, pepper, and oregano. Then roll the sliced veggies in the batter and fry in organic canola oil or safflower oil. You won't believe how delicious they are!

Quick Meals at Home

I know how overwhelming cooking can be when you have a family and a job and a million competing commitments. Luckily, you don't have to sacrifice your kids' health to save time. My cookbook, *The Imus Ranch: Cooking for Kids and Cowboys*, has recipes for great meals that can serve three or thirty. The best part is, most don't take more than a few minutes to prepare.

Avocado, Raspberry, and Mango Salad

The smooth avocado, crunchy nuts, and sweet fruits in this salad offer a terrific combination of flavors and textures.

Preparation time: 15 minutes

4 cups mesclun salad mix

2 cups spinach leaves

2 avocados, peeled, pitted, and diced

¼ cup Imus Ranch Honey-Dijon Dressing (see below)

1 cup fresh raspberries

1 mango, peeled and diced

¼ cup Mr. Martin's Maple-Glazed Pecans (see page 236)

Combine the mesclun and spinach in a large bowl. Add the avocados and dressing and toss gently to combine. Transfer to a serving dish and top with the raspberries, mango, and pecans. Serve with additional dressing on the side, if you like. Makes 4 servings.

Imus Ranch Honey-Dijon Dressing

We use sunflower or safflower oil in many of our dressings because they are monounsaturated—meaning that they help to keep the arteries supple and lubricated—as well as being high in linoleic acid, an essential fatty acid that is one of the major building blocks of the immune system.

Preparation time: 5 minutes

¼ cup honey

⅓ cup balsamic vinegar

3 tablespoons Dijon mustard

1 organic egg or 2 tablespoons liquid egg substitute

½ cup olive oil

½ cup sunflower or safflower oil

1 tablespoon salt

½ teaspoon freshly ground black pepper

Combine the honey, vinegar, mustard, and egg in the container of a food processor and process 1 to 2 minutes. With the motor running, slowly add the oils through the feed tube until the dressing is thickened and well blended. If it seems too thick, add a small amount of water to thin it. Add salt and pepper. Makes 1½ cups.

Andy's Avocado Burger Melt

These delicious sandwiches make perfect weeknight meals. Store-bought veggie burgers come in so many brands and flavors—you can find a lot of variations and never feel as if you've eaten the same burger twice.

Preparation time: 20 minutes
Cooking Time: 13 minutes

2 tablespoons olive oil

½ medium red onion, thinly sliced

4 vegetarian burgers (making your own are the best)

8 slices sourdough bread, toasted

2 to 4 tablespoons Dijon mustard

3 ounces soy Monterey Jack cheese (soy or dairy), sliced

3 large plum tomatoes, thinly sliced

1 avocado, thinly sliced

Heat the oil in a large skillet over medium-high heat. When the oil is shimmering, add the onion and sauté until tender, about 5 minutes. Remove the onion from the pan, reduce the heat to medium low, and add the burgers. Cook, turning once, for 8 minutes, or until golden brown. Spread the toast with the mustard. Top four of the toast slices with burgers, then cheese, tomato, avocado, and sautéed onion. Top with the remaining slices of toast, cut in half, and serve warm. Makes 4 sandwiches.

Recommended Reading

General Health

YOU: The Owner's Manual: An Insider's Guide to the Body That Will Make You Healthier and Younger by Michael F. Roizen and Mehmet Oz is a fun, entertaining introduction to the inner workings of our bodies. A follow-up book, *YOU: On a Diet,* goes into more detail about the importance of eating healthy.

The Checklist: What You and Your Family Need to Know to Prevent Disease and Live a Long and Healthy Life by Manny Alvarez goes decade by decade through a person's development, focusing on the most common health ailments and proactive ways we can prevent them.

Reclaiming Our Health: Exploding the Medical Myth and Embracing the Source of True Healing by John Robbins questions the efficacy of our high-tech approach to medicine and uncovers some of the conflicts of interest present in the mainstream medical community. In this solution-oriented book, Robbins also discusses many important issues related to fertility, childbirth, and women's health in general.

Preconception and Pregnancy

Our Stolen Future: Are We Threatening Our Fertility, Intelligence, and Survival? (www.ourstolenfuture.org), by Theo Colborn, Dianne Dumanoski, and John Peterson Myers. This groundbreaking work brought to the public's attention the role of endocrine disruptors in fetal development, as well as the role of other contaminants in human fertility problems.

For a comprehensive guide to all you can do to detoxify before pregnancy, visit the website www.babieswithouttoxins.org. It contains some great research on the impact of chemicals on the developing fetus, as well as some invaluable tips on detoxification prior to pregnancy.

The book *Detoxify or Die* by Sherry Rogers is another useful resource if you're interested in learning more about the dangerous toxins that might affect your ability to reproduce—and more. Dr. Rogers pinpoints the reasons for the rising incidence of disease in our society and offers ways to reverse the patterns.

The Complete Organic Pregnancy by Deirdre Dolan and Alexandra Zissu also has some great tips on minimizing your exposure to toxins that might harm your future baby. As soon as you decide to make the leap to motherhood, you should consider keeping a few books like this around.

For a natural approach to getting pregnant, check out Toni Weschler's classic *Taking Charge of Your Fertility*. It has a lot of great information about menstruation, pregnancy, and natural birth control.

Christiane Northrup's *Women's Bodies, Women's Wisdom* offers guidance on a vast range of topics relating to women's health: contraceptive methods, fertility at every age, birthing options, and many other subjects. A great encyclopedia of information.

Sandra Steingraber's *Having Faith: An Ecologist's Journey to Motherhood* is an incredible book that explores many of the challenges parents-to-be today face before and during pregnancy. Another must-have resource by Steingraber is *Living Downstream: A Scientist's Personal Investigation of*

Cancer and the Environment. This book is as revolutionary as Rachel Carson's *Silent Spring* was when it was first published in 1962.

The Continuum Concept: In Search of Happiness Lost by Jean Liedloff is another book I highly recommend. Liedloff evaluates Western society and human nature through the lens of the Stone Age Indians she spent two and a half years observing in the jungles of Venezuela.

Life Before Birth: The Challenges of Fetal Development by Peter Nathanielsz can be a little technical at times, but it has a lot of great information on toxins and pregnancy.

Super Baby by Sarah Brewer provides excellent tips for boosting your child's intelligence while he's still in the womb.

Diet and Nutrition

The Complete Organic Pregnancy has a lot of great information about organic food. For tips on natural health, nutrition, and the benefits of organic food, go to www.mambosprouts.com. You'll also find lots of coupons to take with you to the store. Both your body *and* your wallet will be rewarded for your healthier choices at the supermarket!

Marion Nestle's *What to Eat* is an incredible how-to guide to food buying and eating. This wonderful resource explores why we eat what we do and how we can make more thoughtful, nourishing choices.

Disease-Proof Your Child: Feeding Kids Right by Joel Fuhrman. Dr. Fuhrman also has a Web site with lots of useful information about eating right (www.diseaseproof.com).

Vegetarian Baby and *Vegetarian Children: A Supportive Guide for Parents*, both by Sharon Yntema, gave me great information on raising Wyatt vegetarian on a plant-based diet. These books have a lot of useful information on vegetarian lifestyles.

Fast Food Nation by Eric Schlosser gives a horrifying up-close glimpse of the fast-food industry in this country. Before you buy your children their next Happy Meal, read this compelling book. Schlosser, along with Charles

Wilson, also wrote a version of *Fast Food Nation* tailored especially for teens. *Chew on This: Everything You Don't Want to Know About Fast Food* offers a kid-friendly take on the fast-food industry.

The China Study: The Most Comprehensive Study of Nutrition Ever Conducted and the Startling Implications for Diet, Weight Loss, and Long-Term Health by T. Colin Campbell reports on the path-breaking study that established definitive links between nutrition and a variety of diseases, including diabetes, heart diseases, and even cancer. It's not a cookbook, but it does contain a wealth of specific information about why you should eat certain foods and avoid others.

Animal, Vegetable, Miracle: A Year of Food Life by the novelist Barbara Kingsolver describes a year of eating only food that she and her family grew or raised themselves. A really great read.

Cookbooks

The Best-Ever Vegetarian Cookbook by Nicola Graimes truly lives up to its name. A must-have for every parent.

Moosewood Restaurant Simple Suppers by the Moosewood Collective, the subtitle of which is "Fresh Ideas for the Weeknight Table," has easy recipes for pasta, beans, tofu, and main-dish salads.

Vegetarian Suppers from Deborah Madison's Kitchen has recipes for everything from quick, one-dish meals to more elaborate fare. In general, Madison's books have good information on food and its source and the importance of eating locally grown organic foods.

The Candle Cafe Cookbook: More than 150 Enlightened Recipes from New York's Renowned Vegan Restaurant by Joy Pierson, Bart Potenza, and Barbara Scott-Goodman is a testimony to all the delicious dining options available to vegans out there.

SuperFoods HealthStyle: Proven Strategies for Lifelong Health by Steven G. Pratt and Kathy Matthews goes down the list of the "superfoods" that you need to live your fullest life.

Vegetables by James Peterson is a comprehensive guide to buying, storing, and of course preparing sixty-four different vegetables.

Environmental Toxins

Raising Healthy Children in a Toxic World: 101 Smart Solutions for Every Family by Phil Landrigan, Herbert Needleman, and Mary Landrigan is an absolutely essential book, with a ton of practical suggestions for safeguarding your kids from environmental toxins.

The Road to Immunity: How to Survive and Thrive in a Toxic World by Kenneth Bock also explains how you can protect your children, and yourself, from the toxins that are so pervasive in our environment.

Environment California has a great Shopper's Guide to Toxic-Free Kids that's available for download: http://www.environmentcalifornia.org/uploads/B0/av/B0avehMELtJWs0ZmzXiK4w/Shoppers_Guide.pdf.

Holistic Moms (www.holisticmoms.org) hosts a wonderful online community for parents who've decided to raise their children the natural, holistic way.

Green Building and Renovating

Because green building has become so popular in recent years, you can now find extensive resources on any aspect of the subject that interests you. My environmental center's Web site (www.dienviro.com) has extensive, and constantly updated, information on green building. The Green Building Resource Guide (http://greenguide.com) has many useful resources on green building. Or you can go to your local bookstore and browse the offerings before choosing the title or titles that appeal to you most. The following are just a few examples of the many great green-building books now available.

General Green Building

- *Green Remodeling: Changing the World One Room at a Time* by David Johnston and Kim Master

- *Your Green Home: A Guide to Planning a Healthy, Environmentally Friendly New Home* by Alex Wilson

- *Good Green Homes* by Jennifer Roberts

- *The New Ecological Home: A Complete Guide to Green Building Options* by Dan Chiras

- *Natural Remodeling for the Not-So-Green House: Bringing Your Home into Harmony with Nature* by Carol Venolia, Kelly Lerner, and Sarah Susanka

Green Kitchens

- *The Green Kitchen Handbook: Practical Advice, References, and Sources for Transforming the Center of Your Home into a Healthy, Livable Place* by Annie Berthold-Bond

- *Good Green Kitchens* by Jennifer Roberts

"Green" Pediatrics

The American Academy of Pediatrics has published an accompaniment to its famed Red Book, called *Pediatric Environmental Health* (second edition), which we refer to as the "Green Book." While this book is by no means as comprehensive as many green pediatricians would like, this handbook, which was first published in 1999, does represent real progress on the part of the mainstream medical establishment. While written to help pediatricians recognize various environmental threats to their young patients' health, parents would benefit from familiarizing themselves with its contents, too. You can buy this essential text on the AAP's Web site (www.aap.org/bst/showdetl.cfm?&DID=15&Product_ID=1697).

General Homeopathy

For basic information on the principles of homeopathy, visit the federal government's National Center for Complementary and Alternative Medicine's Web site (www.nccam.nih.gov), which gives an overview of this branch of alternative medicine. You can also access fact sheets about a wide range of dietary supplements and the individual herbs used in various homeopathic formulas.

Homeopathic Medicine for Children and Infants by Dana Ullman and *Homeopathic Medicine at Home: Natural Remedies for Everyday Ailments and Minor Injuries* by Maesimund B. Panos and Jane Heimlich are both great resources for parents interested in learning more about the centuries-old principles of homeopathy.

Alternative Cures: The Most Effective Natural Home Remedies for 160 Health Problems by Bill Gottlieb offers a huge range of easy, drug-free solutions for a wide range of medical complaints, providing relief from everything from asthma to anxiety.

Back to Eden by Jethro Kloss is a classic guide to herbal medicine. Originally published in 1939, Kloss's book promotes the benefits of an organic, whole-foods diet and a holistic approach to health. Kloss was a visionary, and many of his lessons are still relevant, and powerful, today.

Quantum Healing by Deepak Chopra explores the fundamental principles of mind-body healing and helps explain how the body can heal itself. An abridged version of this text is also available on audiotape.

Prescription for Nutritional Healing: A Practical A-to-Z Reference to Drug-Free Remedies Using Vitamins, Minerals, Herbs and Food Supplements by nutritionist Phyllis A. Balch and doctor James F. Balch, M.D., is another must-have resource that you can find at Whole Foods.

Infant Massage

Nurse Karen Overgaard, who works with my environmental center at Hackensack, recommended these books on infant massage, which she and other prominent "green" health-care providers, including Dr. Lawrence Rosen, recommend for reducing stress in both infants and parents.

- *Baby Massage: The Calming Power of Touch* by Alan Heath and Nicki Bainbridge
- *The Fussy Baby* by Dr. William Sears
- *The Vital Touch* by Sharon Heller
- *Touch* by Tiffany Field

Nurse Karen recommends using cold-pressed oils (such as grapeseed oil) or calendula baby oil from Weleda.

Reiki

The Power of Reiki by Tanmaya Honervogt shows many different hand positions.

An Introduction to Reiki by Mary Lambert and Chris Parkes gives a great overview of the 2,500-year-old principles of Reiki. It also demonstrates hand positions and other basics of this healing art.

Pet Care

To take care of your baby properly, you need to make sure that you're keeping toxins away from your pets as well. Kristen Leigh Bell has written an extremely useful book on holistic pet care, *Holistic Aromatherapy for*

Animals. C.J. Puotinen's *Natural Remedies for Cats and Dogs* is also a good reference.

Essential Oils

My favorite book on essential oils, Dr. Young's *Essential Oils Desk Reference,* contains all sorts of information on the therapeutic benefits of essential oils and the specific properties of individual oils.

Dr. Gary Young's *Essential Oils Integrative Medical Guide: Building Immunity, Increasing Longevity, and Enhancing Mental Performance with Therapeutic-Grade Essential Oils* goes into more detail about which oils to use for specific health problems.

Specific Health Disorders

In *Autism, Brain, and Environment*, Richard Lathe attributes the recent increase in cases of autism to a combination of genetic predisposition and environmental toxins. This book is worth reading if you want to learn more about autism and what causes it. For more information on the vaccination-autism debate, visit the Web site of my environmental center (www.dienviro.com), SafeMinds (www.safeminds.org), the National Autism Association (www.nationalautismassociation.org), and Generation Rescue (www.generationrescue.org).

Natural Relief for Your Child's Asthma: A Guide to Controlling Symptoms and Reducing Your Child's Dependence on Drugs by Stephen Bock, Kenneth Bock, and Nancy Bruning is an excellent resource for parents seeking a holistic approach to treating their children's asthma.

Healing the New Childhood Epidemics: Autism, ADHD, Asthma, and Allergies: The Groundbreaking Program for the 4-A Disorders by Kenneth Bock and Cameron Stauth investigates the root cause of these childhood epidemics and offers innovative healing solutions.

Children with Starving Brains: A Medical Treatment Guide for Au-

tism Spectrum Disorder by Jaquelyn McCandless goes into detail about the causes of ASDs and offers innovative, effective treatment options.

The Cure for All Cancers: Including over 100 Case Histories of Persons Cured by Hulda Regehr Clark outlines a revolutionary protocol for not just treating, but curing, cancer. Clark has also written a book called *The Cure for All Diseases* that addresses other serious chronic illnesses.

Education

You Are Your Child's First Teacher: What Parents Can Do with and for Their Children from Birth to Age Six by Rahima Baldwin Dancy offers an easy-to-apply adaptation of Rudolf Steiner's approach to childhood development. Dancy's clear, concise writing offers parents a holistic approach to children's physical, emotional, psychological, spiritual, and intellectual selves.

Childhood, A Study of the Growing Child by Caroline von Heydebrand focuses on the spiritual development of the child and the development of consciousness.

Leisure

Toymaking with Children by Freya Jaffke offers suggestions for age-appropriate toys and instructions for toys you and your child can make together at home.

Buying Green: A Web Reference Guide

Even if you live in a rural area, you can find just about any of these products on the Web. But remember, even if you're buying products online, make sure you know what's in them. You want to avoid clothing treated with pesticides; toys made with lead and PVCs; personal-care products that contain petroleum distillates, parabens, sulfates, and propylene glycol; and household cleaners that contain chlorine bleach and ammonia.

Green Cleaning

Greening your cleaning is the simplest—and most essential—step you can take to clean up your family's indoor environment.

- Imus's Greening the Cleaning institutional and retail product line. One hundred percent of the after-tax profits from sales of my products go to the Imus Cattle Ranch for Kids with Cancer. You can purchase products from my retail line—laundry liquid, hand dishwashing liquid, Citrus Sage All-Purpose Cleaner, Citrus Sage Glass and Window Cleaner—at www.imusranch foods.com and at thousands of stores all over the country.

- Biokleen (www.biokleenhome.com)

- Ecover (www.ecover.com)

- Earth Friendly Products (www.ecos.com)

- Seventh Generation (www.seventhgeneration.com)

- Sun and Earth (www.sunandearth.com)

- Planet (www.planetinc.com)

Green Building

Green building is getting easier and more affordable every day. Visit my Web site (www.dienviro.com) for a wide range of suggestions. We frequently update the green-building information.

Flooring: All of these companies offer some excellent green flooring choices:

- Armstrong (www.armstrong.com)

- Beaulieu of America (www.beaulieu-usa.com)

- Carpet America Recovery Effort (www.carpetrecovery.org)

- Colin Campbell and Sons (www.colcam.com)

- Earth Weave Carpet Mills (www.earthweave.com)

- Mannington (www.mannington.com)

- Rivanna Natural Designs (www.rivannadesigns.com)

For information on specific flooring materials, refer to these Web sites:

- Building Green (cork) (www.buildinggreen.com/products/cork_flooring.cfm)

- Environmental Bamboo Foundation (bamboo) (www
  .bamboocentral.org)
- Forest Stewardship Council (wood) (www.fscus.org)
- Green Home (linoleum) (www.greeenhome.com)

Water Filtration

If you're thinking of installing a water-filtration system in your home, you should visit several informative Web sites that allow you to compare different systems and see which one is right for your family.

- **Water Filter Comparisons** (www.waterfiltercomparisons .net) is an excellent site that lists many of the filters out there for the home and explains what different filters remove from the water. Some just filter out chlorine and lead, while others filter out lindane, VOCs, and other contaminants. Among the filters compared are Aquasana, Amway, Culligan, Kenmore, GE, Pūr, and Brita.

- **The Consumer Search** Web site (www.consumersearch .net) compares all the different types of filtration systems out there and ranks them according to efficacy. Categories include the best pitcher filter, the best horizontal filter, the best under-the-sink filter, the best faucet filter, and so on.

- Other useful Web sites include www.thebestwaterfilters .com, www.bestfilters.com, www.freedrinkingwater.com, and www.h2owarehouse.com.

Toys

Purchasing safe, nontoxic toys isn't as difficult as it sounds, or not anymore. As more and more parents learn about the dangers of these toys, they're demanding safer alternatives. As a result, many companies are acting to limit PVC and phthalate use in the toys they manufacture, and environmentally friendly toys are becoming easier to find all the time. These companies all make great nontoxic toys that your kids will love:

- Hugg-A-Planet (www.peacetoys.com)

- Lego (www.lego.com)

- Island Treasure Toys (www.islandtreasuretoys.com) makes toys for creative children, including play silks, wooden toys, dolls, games, and wooden play food.

- Baby Bunz & Co. (www.babybunz.com)

- Baby Mine Store (www.BabyMineStore.com)

- Brio (http://brio.knex.com)

- Guidecraft (www.guidecraft.com)

- HearthSong (www.hearthsong.com) has excellent educational toys, craft kits, and more for kids of all ages.

- Imaginarium Toys (www.imaginarium.com), a division of Toys "R" Us, makes wooden toys, art supplies, craft kits, musical instruments, and other educational toys.

- Lakeshore Learning Store (www.lakeshorelearning.com) has a huge selection of wooden toys, art supplies, cloth dolls, craft kits, books, CDs, musical instruments, and other developmental toys from birth through grade eight. It also has great catalogs and online resources.

- Little Tikes (www.littletikes.com)

- Mercurius (www.mercurius-usa.com)

- Natural Play (www.NaturalPlay.com)

- Nova Natural Toys and Crafts (www.novanatural.com). Wholesale Nova Toys sells a selection of toys, some with quantity requirements (Phone: 1-877-356-8671)

- Plan Toys (www.plantoys.com) are great.

- Primetime Playthings (www.intplay.com)

- Sassy (www.sassybaby.com)

- Tiny Love (www.tinylove.com)

- Viking Toys

Personal-Care Products

- California Baby (www.californiababy.com) makes our favorite bubble bath.

- Weleda (www.usa.weleda.com) makes great organic personal-care products for babies and new mothers.

- Aubrey Organics (www.aubrey-organics.com) offers a wide selection of natural and organic lotions and shampoos. When Wyatt was a baby, I frequently used Aubrey Organics shampoos on him.

- Erbaviva (www.erbaviva.com) also makes various safe, nontoxic products for babies and mothers.

Sun Protection

- California Baby Everyday/Year-Round Moisturizing Sunscreen Lotion, SPF 18 (www.californiababy.com)

- Weleda Children's Sunscreen, SPF 18+ (www.usa.weleda.com)

- Aubrey Organics Natural Sun Green Tea Protective Sunscreen, SPF 25 (www.aubrey-organics.com)

- Kiss My Face Sunspray Lotion, SPF 30 (www.kissmyface.com)

- Erbaviva Children's Sunscreen, SPF 15 (www.erbaviva.com)

- All Terrain (www.allterrainco.com) makes natural sunscreen and bug spray.

Clothing

- Maggie's Functional Organics (www.maggiesorganics.com) makes great organic clothing for babies and adults.

- Cozy Cocoon (www.cozycocoon.com) makes beautiful swaddling outfits.

- The Gaiam catalog (www.gaiam.com) is an excellent resources for organic clothing for mother and baby alike, as well as organic bedding, safe toys, and various other lifestyle accessories.

- Whole Foods is another place to find organic cotton clothing at extremely reasonable prices. The selection might not be as extensive as in some of these online catalogs, but for people who live near a Whole Foods, the convenience can't be beat.

Important Legislation

Many of these bills would never even have been introduced without the support of parents like you and me. While several important bills have been passed in recent years, we have more work to do on the legislative level for our kids. To bring these important changes to your community, write or email your congressman. You can find your representative's contact details by visiting www.house.gov/

Kid Safe Chemicals Act: There are 82,000 chemicals currently in use in the United States, most of which have not been tested for safety. In the thirty-nine years since the Toxic Substances Control Act was passed in 1976, the EPA has banned or restricted the use of only five chemical substances. This bill proposes to amend the Toxic Substances Control Act to reduce the exposure of kids, workers, and consumers to toxic chemicals and to require more stringent and effective testing for chemicals used in consumer products. Senator Frank Lautenberg of New Jersey is sponsoring this bill, which requires all chemicals used in the home to be evaluated for their safety on children. It also mandates that companies list any ingredients in their products that are mutagens, teratogens, endocrine or hormone disrupters, neurotoxins, or carcinogens.

Combating Autism Act of 2006: The Senate unanimously passed this crucial piece of legislation on August 3, 2006, and President Bush signed it into law four months later. The historic passage of this bill—which will increase federal spending on autism and autism spectrum disorders (ASDs) by nearly 50 percent—represents a real call to action on the part of our government.

Conquer Childhood Cancer Act of 2007: This act amends the Public Health Service Act to advance our knowledge and treatment of pediatric cancers.

Lead-Free Toys Act: First introduced in 2005, this bill received widespread attention after the lead-toy scare during the summer of 2007. It would require the Consumer Product Safety commission to ban any children's product containing lead under the Hazardous Substances Act. At the moment, there are no federal limits on lead in children's products, unless they contain lead paint, in which case they're regulated under the lead-in-paint law.

Mercury-Free Vaccine Legislation: Across the country, individual states are taking a stand against manufacturing vaccines with the preservative thimerosal. Important changes are also taking place on the national level. The Mercury-Free Vaccines Act of 2005 amends the federal Food, Drug, and Cosmetic Act to designate a banned mercury-containing vaccine as adulterated. It also amends the Public Health Service Act to stipulate that a vaccine is banned if it contains 1 or more micrograms of mercury per dose.

Comprehensive Comparative Study of Vaccinated and Unvaccinated Populations Act of 2007: This bill would require the NIH to conduct a comprehensive study to compare total health outcomes, including the risk of autism, between vaccinated and unvaccinated U.S. populations and also to determine whether vaccines or vaccine components play a role in the development of autism spectrum disorder or other neurological conditions.

Studies on Children's Health

In addition to rallying for the passage of better laws, we also need to put pressure on the government to devote more resources to studying the impact of the environment on children's health. All over the country, researchers and experts are connecting the dots on a number of issues, but there's still so much more that we need to learn in order to protect our children.

The National Children's Study

In September of 2005, the National Institute of Child Health and Human Development outlined an ambitious plan to assess the impact of the environment on childhood health. By studying the environmental exposures of one hundred thousand children throughout the country, the creators of the National Children's Study are determined to isolate the root cause of many common childhood conditions and disorders, including asthma, premature birth, birth defects, heart disease, leukemia, diabetes, autism, dyslexia, mental retardation, ADHD, and obesity.

By tracking these one hundred thousand children from conception to age twenty-one, the National Children's Study will be addressing one of the major problems the scientific and medical establishments are facing today: Even as we're getting better at treating these diseases, in the vast majority of cases we still don't know what's causing them.

The connections between environmental exposures and childhood diseases, Dr. Phil Landrigan said, "are just beginning to appear out of the mist." The National Children's Study is designed to give doctors, researchers, and parents a better understanding of these connections. "Knowledge is power," Dr. Landrigan said. "If we understand the risks [our children are facing], then we can do something about it." In other words: The more we learn about what's causing these diseases, the more we'll be able to prevent them.

"The goal of the study," Dr. Landrigan said, "is to identify and to characterize all the factors in the environment that influence children's health, their development, and their risk of disease—to detect associations between exposures and disease."

The National Children's Study offers our best hope of getting this cause-and-effect information. It will study children from every region of the country and every segment of the population. And it will study them before they get sick, not after, like so many previous studies.

"We're going to look at toxic chemicals; we're going to look at the home environment. We're going to look at social factors in the environment; we're going to look at the communities in which these one hundred thousand children grow up. And we're going to be measuring the impact of exposures on children's health. And the way we're going to measure these exposures is by enrolling families in the study right at the beginning of pregnancy."

And, in an effort to learn more about how genes interact with the environment, National Children's Study researchers will take the child's whole history into account and track every stage of his or her development. "We'll take a very careful history from the mother and from the father, about all their exposures," Dr. Landrigan said. "We'll take biological samples, we'll take blood, we'll take urine, we'll take hair from the mom, to measure all the chemicals that were in her body that might influence the health of the baby. When the baby is born, we'll take a sample of blood from the umbilical cord, we'll take a sample of the placenta. We'll do a careful examination of the baby. And during the pregnancy, we will have looked at the baby through a very systematic ultrasound examination, and then do a newborn exam. And then at six months, twelve months, twenty-four months, thirty-six months, and so on, we'll do very careful physicals, very careful developmental assessments on each child in the study, so we can see how the child is doing."

We can't wait much longer to launch this essential study. With so many of our children suffering, we desperately need to learn more about the root cause of these diseases and what we can do to prevent them. The timing is right in every respect. "Over the last twenty-five years," Dr. Landrigan said, "we've learned how to do these big studies. We have the Framingham Heart Study, Women's Health Initiative, and a bunch of other big, multiyear, multicenter studies." We've also developed the know-how, and the technology, to run these studies efficiently. "We can now measure hundreds of chemicals in blood and urine down to very low levels," said Dr. Landrigan. This marvelous technology, didn't exist even five or ten years ago.

Another reason to do the study now is that "we've decoded the human genome. We can now measure the DNA of the mother and the father and the baby. We can identify the different genes that are present in them, and we can look for the interplay between the environmental exposures and the genes. Everybody's different. Different people react differently to different chemicals. And by knowing both the chemicals and the genes, we can map all that out."

You might be thinking: Fine. This is all very interesting, but what does the National Children's Study have to do with me? Well, if your child has ever been diagnosed with an illness, you probably had a lot of questions for your pediatrician. You probably wanted to know why your kid was sick and if you could've done anything to prevent it.

For many of these diseases, doctors can't provide satisfactory explanations—not even close. Dr. Landrigan offered the example of a five-year-old child diagnosed with autism. If a doctor wants to determine which environmental exposures might have triggered the autism, what can he do? "You go to these poor parents who are suffering with the autistic kid, and you say to them, 'What were you exposed to when you were pregnant?' And they have an hour. Well, it was five years ago." It's just not acceptable that such crucial information should be left to faulty memories and desperate guesswork. The stakes are just too high.

The National Children's Study works differently. It's a prospective study, which Dr. Landrigan explained means that "it will enroll the babies before they're even born and then follow them prospectively in real time, as they grow up.

"And the reason that's so important," he said, "is that we will measure their exposures before any illness occurs. We'll be getting those blood samples on the mom during pregnancy; we'll be getting the cord blood at birth; we'll be getting blood and urine samples from the children as they grow up. And then all those analyses will be done; samples will be put in the deep freeze, so we can measure other stuff that we haven't thought of yet. And the measurements are going to be made completely separate from any assessment of disease in the kids."

In the future, the National Children's Study will clarify the relationship between childhood diseases and environmental exposures, for doctors and parents. Parents with sick kids will no longer wonder what they did wrong, or agonize over different choices they might have made. At this stage, we lack so much crucial knowledge. There are too many question marks and what-ifs. We need answers—answers that only the National Children's Study can provide.

In 2007, the Congress approved $69 million to fund the National Children's Study. Many other environmental organizations, like the National Institute of Environmental Health Sciences and the Centers for Disease Control, are contributing as well.

Sounds like a lot of money, right? Well, consider this: Treating childhood cancer alone costs our society an estimated $600 million every year. The total cost of treating childhood diseases caused by environmental insults is an amazing $54.9 billion every year—that's approximately 2.8 percent of total health care costs!

The National Children's Study operates on a tiny fraction of this unbelievable figure. It just makes common sense that investing in our children's future today will in the long run save us a tremendous amount, of both money and heartache. In other words, we can't afford not to do this study. Write to your local congressional representative about the necessity of protecting this study. For too long, children's health has not ranked among our top priorities, and as a society, we're beginning to suffer the consequences.

Countries all over the world are coming together to recognize the importance of these studies, Dr. Landrigan told me. The World Health Organization, he said, "is in the process of launching studies like the National Children's Study in ten or fifteen more countries, ranging from Thailand to Western Europe. And to the extent possible, we're using the same protocols in these various studies, so the information will be comparable."

He went on: "We hope that in a few years' time, we can begin to do comparisons across countries, and in some cases maybe even link the data. And if we can link the information—if we can take one hundred thousand kids from Sweden and one hundred thousand from Italy and put them with one hundred thousand from the United States, and pool the information to look, for example, at childhood cancer—that's an incredibly powerful study. The benefits for protecting children's health will be truly enormous."

Mothers and Newborns Study

Researchers like Dr. Frederica Perera, who directs the Center for Children's Environmental Health at Columbia University, are conducting smaller-scale studies linking childhood disease to environmental exposures. "We know cancer involves accumulating genetic changes that manifest in adulthood," she told me, citing one example of a disease that's caused by an interaction of genes with the environment. "That process starts in the womb, much earlier than anyone would've thought. There's a special risk at that early stage of development," she said. "We're trying to understand this window of vulnerability. That's what this study concentrates on: the sustained effects that manifest themselves from this moment up to adolescence."

In an effort to understand more about these "windows of vulnerability," Perera's center has launched the Mothers and Newborns in New York City Study, which examines the chronic exposures of pregnant women in the low-income Manhattan neighborhoods of Harlem, Washington Heights, and the South Bronx.

"We've enrolled 730 mothers in the study," she said. "For two days, they wear a backpack that measures things around them, which gives us a pretty good snapshot of what's to come. We find out whether they have medium, low, or high exposure to toxins in the air. We also collect urine and the baby's first bowel movement, and we analyze biomarkers in those. The mother is being exposed to things in the air and in her diet—we measure dose, damage, and genetic expression. Then, the babies are brought in at three months, six months, and at one year. Our oldest children in the study are now eight."

The Mothers and Newborns Study primarily focuses on prenatal development, for one simple reason. "Because it is growing so quickly, the fetus has tremendous potential for damage," Perera said. "Damage to the fetus is ten times higher than that to the mother at the exact same unit of exposure or dose. Mercury and lead, for example, have *much* greater effect at this stage than later on. The fetus lacks the systems to detoxify and repair DNA. By being more vigilant during this prenatal stage, we've had a greater effect." The study has already established links between prenatal exposures to air pollutants and pesticides and reduced fetal growth. But, Perera adds, "measuring medical and developmental disorders over time" is extremely expensive and requires a great deal of staff. The National Children's Study (see page 256) aims to study these same factors on a much broader scale, by following a much wider cross-section of children from preconception to adulthood.

For more information on the studies conducted by Perera and her colleagues at Columbia, refer to www.ccceh.org.

I'm not citing these studies and statistics to frighten you—on the contrary. We can't control every single factor that influences our children's health, but we're by no means powerless. If we work together, we can reduce the concentration of chemicals our children are exposed to before birth. By educating ourselves, and controlling our toxic exposures, we can make all the difference in the health of future generations. As parents, we have a responsibility to fight for more research like Perera's.

Studies on Mercury Toxicity and Autism

Over the last few years, numerous studies have shown how mercury exposure in early childhood could be contributing to the rise of autism and other developmental disorders. A 2004 Columbia Univerisity study reported behavioral characteristics in immune-compromised mice injected with thimerosal that appear similar to autism. Another significant study from the University of Arkansas found that many autistic children are genetically deficient in their ability to produce glutathione, an antioxidant produced in the brain that helps remove mercury from the body. Urinary porphyrin studies confirm that many autistic children have much higher than normal concentrations of mercury in their bodies.

In 2007, Generation Rescue (www.generationrescue.org), a parent-led organization, released the findings of its independent study comparing vaccinated and unvaccinated children in nine counties in Oregon and

California. Using the same formula as the CDC, the study determined that vaccinated children were two and a half times more likely to have neurological disorders like autism and ADHD.

Most parents didn't hear about this study, just as they didn't hear about the 2006 study that demonstrated that small amounts of thimerosal, smaller than what is found in one influenza vaccine, can damage the immune system.

Glossary of Environmental Health Terms

The majority of these definitions have been adopted from the glossary of terms published by the Agency for Toxic Substances and Disease Registry.

Absorption: How a chemical enters a person's blood after the chemical has been swallowed, has come into contact with the skin, or has been breathed in.

Acute exposure: Contact with a chemical that happens once or only for a limited period of time. ATSDR defines acute exposures as those that might last up to fourteen days.

Additive effect: A response to a chemical mixture, or combination of substances, that might be expected if the known effects of individual chemicals, seen at specific doses, were added together.

Adverse health effect: A change in body function or the structures of cells that can lead to disease or health problems.

ATSDR: The Agency for Toxic Substances and Disease Registry. ATSDR is a federal health agency in Atlanta, Georgia, that deals with hazardous substance and waste-site issues. ATSDR gives people information about harmful chemicals in their environment and tells people how to protect themselves from coming into contact with such chemicals.

Cancer: A group of diseases that occur when cells in the body become abnormal and grow, or multiply, out of control.

Carcinogen: Any substance shown to cause tumors or cancer in experimental studies. Response, Compensation, and Liability Act.

Chronic exposure: A contact with a substance or chemical that happens over a long period of time. ATSDR considers exposures of more than one year to be chronic.

Completed exposure pathway: See *Exposure pathway*.

Concentration: How much or the amount of a substance present in a certain amount of soil, water, air, or food.

Contaminant: See *Environmental contaminant*.

Delayed health effect: A disease or injury that results from exposures that may have occurred far in the past.

Dermal contact: A chemical getting onto your skin. (See also *Route of exposure*.)

Dose: The amount of a substance to which a person may be exposed, usually on a daily basis. Dose is often quantified as the "amount of substance(s) per body weight per day."

Dose/response: The relationship between the amount of exposure (dose) and the change in body function or health that results from it.

Duration: The amount of time (days, months, years) that a person is exposed to a chemical.

Endocrine disruptor: An endocrine disruptor is any substance that can interfere with natural hormones. Exposure to these chemicals could disrupt the body's hormone signals that regulate reproduction and development, either by blocking or mimicking the action of hormones. In men, endocrine disruptors can lead to reduced sperm counts and undescended testicles. Endocrine disruptors are also associated with endometriosis, altered immune function, and developmental disabilities.

Environmental contaminant: A substance (chemical) that gets into a system (person, animal, or the environment) in amounts higher than the expected or naturally occurring levels in a specific environment.

Environmental Protection Agency (EPA): The U.S. federal agency that develops and enforces environmental laws to protect the environment and the public's health.

Epidemiology: The study of the incidence, distribution, and control of disease.

Estrogen mimic: Estrogen mimics are chemicals that our bodies perceive to be estrogen. Estrogen is a naturally occurring hormone that governs the development of female characteristics. Women have higher levels of estrogen than men. Estrogen mimics pose a threat to human health because our bodies perceive them to be estrogen. Estrogenic toxins enter our bodies through various paths, including through the foods we eat, particularly meat, poultry, and nonorganic high-fat dairy products.

Exposure: Contact with a chemical substance. (For the three ways people can come into contact with substances, see *Route of exposure*.)

Exposure assessment: The process of determining the ways people come in contact with chemicals, the duration and frequency of this contact, and the concentrations of the chemicals involved.

Exposure pathway: A description of the way that a chemical moves from its source to where and how people can come into contact with (or get exposed to) it. ATSDR defines an exposure pathway as having five parts:

1. Source of contamination
2. Environmental media and transport mechanism
3. Point of exposure
4. Route of exposure
5. Receptor population

When all five parts of an exposure pathway are present, it is called a "completed exposure pathway."

Frequency: How often a person is exposed to a chemical over time; for example, every day, once a week, twice a month.

Hazardous waste: Substances that have been released or thrown away into the environment and that, under certain conditions, could be harmful to people who come into contact with them.

Ingestion: Swallowing something, as in eating or drinking. Ingestion is one of three ways a chemical can enter your body. (See also *Route of exposure*.)

Inhalation: Breathing. Inhalation is one of three ways a chemical can enter your body. (See also *Route of exposure*.)

LOAEL (lowest observed adverse effect level): The lowest dose of a chemical in a study, or group of studies, that has caused harmful health effects in people or animals.

MRL (minimal risk level): An estimate of daily human exposure—by a specified route and length of time—to a dose of chemical that is likely to be without a measurable risk of adverse, noncancerous effects. An MRL should *not* be used as a predictor of adverse health effects.

Mutagen: A mutagen is any agent that causes a permanent genetic change in a cell. The term "mutagenicity" refers to the capacity of a chemical or physical agent to bring about this unnatural permanent alteration.

Neurotoxin: A neurotoxin is any poisonous chemical that acts on the body's brain and nervous system. Neurotoxins, which can affect cognitive function, have been linked to reduced IQs in children. Known neurotoxins include formaldehyde (which is also a carcinogen), mercury, and manganese.

Persistent bioaccumulative toxins (PBTs): Compounds that persist in the environment once introduced. A compound may persist for less than a second or indefinitely, for tens or thousands of years. A bioaccumulative substance is one that increases in concentration in living organisms over time. When toxins bioaccumulate in the fatty tissues of our bodies, they can cause serious long-term health problems and even alter our genetic makeup permanently.

Point of exposure: The place where someone can come into contact with a contaminated environmental medium (air, water, food, or soil). These are all examples of points of exposure: a playground with contaminated dirt, a contaminated spring used for drinking water, contaminated soil where fruits or vegetables are grown, or an apartment overlooking a large bus station.

Population: A group of people living in a certain area, or the number of people in a certain area or group.

Receptor population: People who live or work in the path of one or more chemicals and who could come into contact with them. (See also *Exposure pathway*.)

Reference dose (RfD): An estimate, with safety factors (see *Safety factor*) built in, of the daily, life-time exposure of human populations to a possible hazard that is not likely to cause harm to a person.

Route of exposure: The way a chemical can get into a person's body. There are three exposure routes:

1. Breathing (also called inhalation)
2. Eating or drinking (also called ingestion)
3. Skin (or dermal) contact.

Safety factor: Also called the "uncertainty factor." When scientists don't have enough information to decide if an exposure will cause harm to people, they use "safety factors" and formulas in place of the unknown information. These factors and formulas can help determine the amount of a chemical that is not likely to cause harm to people.

Source (of contamination): The place where a chemical comes from, such as a landfill, pond, or incinerator. The contaminant source is the first part of an *Exposure pathway*.

Special populations: People who may be more sensitive to chemical exposures because of specific factors such as age, a preexisting disease, occupation, sex, or certain behaviors (like cigarette smoking). Children, pregnant women, and the elderly are often considered special populations.

Synergistic effect: A health effect from an exposure to more than one chemical, wherein one of the chemicals worsens the effect of another chemical. The combined effect of the chemicals together exceeds the effects of any one chemical in isolation.

Teratogen: Teratogens are substances that interfere with embryonic or fetal development, causing malformation or serious deviation from normal development in the womb.

Toxic: Harmful. Any substance or chemical can be toxic at a certain dose (amount). The dose is what determines the potential harm of a chemical and whether it would cause someone to get sick.

Toxic chemical: Toxic chemicals are substances that can cause severe illness, poisoning, birth defects, disease, or death when ingested, inhaled, or absorbed by living organisms.

Toxic pollutants: Toxic pollutants are materials contaminating the environment that cause death, disease, and birth defects in organisms that ingest or absorb them. The quantities and length of exposure necessary to cause these effects can vary widely.

Toxic Release Inventory (TRI): A database of annual toxic releases from certain manufacturers that must report annually to the EPA, stating the amounts of almost 350 toxic chemicals in 22 chemical categories that they release directly to air, water, or land, inject underground, or transfer to off-site facilities. The EPA compiles these reports and makes the information available to the public under the Community Right-to-Know portion of the law.

Toxic substance: A toxic substance is a chemical or mixture that can cause illness, death, disease, or birth defects. The quantities and exposures necessary to cause these effects can vary widely. Many toxic substances are pollutants and contaminants in the environment.

Toxic waste: Toxic waste is a waste that can produce injury if inhaled, swallowed, or absorbed through the skin.

Toxicology: The study of the harmful effects of chemicals on humans or animals.

Tumor: Abnormal growth of tissue or cells that produces a lump or mass.

Volatile organic compound (VOC): VOCs are substances containing carbon and different proportions of other elements such as hydrogen, oxygen, fluorine, chlorine, bromine, sulfur, or nitrogen; these substances easily become vapor or gases.

Waterborne contaminants are unhealthy chemicals, microorganisms (like bacteria), or radiation found in tap water.

Biographies of Medical Experts

Manuel Alvarez, M.D., is chairman of the Department of Obstetrics and Gynecology and Reproductive Science at Hackensack University Medical Center. He also serves as a FOX News Channel (FNC) medical contributor, appearing primarily on its daytime line-up, which includes *FOX & Friends* and *Dayside*. Known widely to audiences as Dr. Manny, Alvarez was previously a health science reporter for Telemundo and developed a nightly news segment entitled "A Dose of Health.

Dr. Alvarez is also adjunct professor of obstetrics and gynecology at New York University School of Medicine in New York City, as well as visiting professor at Yale School of Medicine in Connecticut. He is certified by the American Board of Obstetrics and Gynecology and is also Board Certified in Maternal Fetal Medicine. Dr. Alvarez is a member of many professional societies including the American College of Obstetricians and Gynecologists, the Society of Prenatal Care and the American Institute of Ultrasound in Medicine. In 2004, Dr. Alvarez was named the Man of the Year by New Jersey SEEDS, an organization that provides educational scholarships for students. Born in Cuba, Dr. Alvarez lives in New Jersey with his wife, Katarina, and their three children, Rex, Ryan, and Olivia. For more information, visit Dr. Alvarez on the web at http://www.askdrmanny.com/ or http://www.foxnews.com/health/index.html.

Frances Beinecke is president of the Natural Resources Defense Council (NRDC). Under her leadership, NRDC has launched major initiatives on global warming, oil dependence, reviving the oceans, saving wild places, stemming the tide of toxic chemicals, and the greening of China. Ms. Beinecke has worked with NRDC for more than thirty years. Prior to becoming president in 2006, she was the organization's executive director for eight years, during which time NRDC's membership doubled and the staff grew to over 300.

Ms. Beinecke has had leadership roles in several other environmental organizations as well, including the World Resources Institute, the Energy Future Coalition, and the Conservation International's Center for Environmental Leadership in Business. She received a bachelor's degree from Yale College and a master's degree from the Yale School of Forestry & Environmental Studies. She co-chairs the Leadership Council of the Yale School of Forestry, is a member of the Yale School of Management's Advisory Board, and a former member of the Yale Corporation. Ms. Beinecke has received the Rachel Carson Award from the National Audubon Society, the Distinguished Alumni Award from Yale, the Annual Conservation Award from the Adirondack Council, and the Robert Marshall Award from the Wilderness Society.

Kenneth A. Bock, M.D., F.A.A.F.P., F.A.C.N., received his medical degree with Honor from the University of Rochester School of Medicine in 1979. He is the co-founder and co-director of the Rhinebeck Health Center, and a clinical instructor in Family Medicine at the Albany Medical College. He is also the author of *The Road to Immunity: How To Survive and Thrive in a Toxic World* and the co-author of *Natural Relief for Your Child's Asthma: A Guide to Controlling Symptoms & Reducing Your Child's Dependence on Drugs* and, most recently, *Healing the New Childhood Epidemics: Autism, ADHD, Asthma and Allergies: The Groundbreaking Program for the 4-A Disorders*. For the past twenty-five years, he has dealt with complex medical problems by integrating alternative modalities with conventional medicine into a comprehensive integrative medical practice, and for the last eight years he has focused that approach on children with autism spectrum disorders, ADHD, asthma, and allergies. Dr. Bock's Healing Program is at the vanguard of the new biomedical approach to the treatment of children affected by these disorders. Dr. Bock lives in Woodstock, New York, with his wife and two children.

Jeffrey R. Boscamp, M.D., is the Marvin I. Gottlieb, M.D., Ph.D. chairman of pediatrics, and physician in chief of the Joseph M. Sanzari Children's Hospital at Hackensack University Medical Center. He is also the founder of the Section of Pediatric Infectious Diseases. He is an associate professor of pediatrics at the UMDNJ–New Jersey Medical School and is also the founder of the Steven Bader Immunologic Institute at Hackensack University Medical Center.

Dr. Boscamp received his B.A. from Williams College and his M.D. from New York Medical College. He completed his pediatric residency at Babies Hospital, Columbia Presbyterian Medical Center, and a fellowship in adult and pediatric infectious diseases at the Albert Einstein College of Medicine.

Dr. Boscamp is chairman of the N.J. Chapter, American Academy of Pediatrics, Committee on Infectious Diseases. His research interests are in immunocompromised children, antibiotics, and Lyme disease, and he is the author of numerous articles and book chapters. He has received several awards for outstanding teaching of medical students and residents. Dr. Boscamp has been a frequent speaker at continuing education programs and national conferences.

Devra Davis, Ph.D., MPH, is director of the Center for Environmental Oncology at the University of Pittsburg Cancer Institute. She's an environmental health expert, a professor of epidemiology at the University of Pittsburg Graduate School of Public Health, and a visiting professor at Carnegie Mellon University's Heinz School of Public Policy and Management. Dr. Davis was designated a National Book Award Finalist for her book *When Smoke Ran Like Water*, and her new book, *The Secret History of the War on Cancer*, is becoming a best-seller in the world of public health. In addition to her academic appointments, Dr. Davis has held multiple advisory roles in national and international agencies, including the World Health Organization, and has received numerous awards pertaining to her work in environmental health. Dr. Davis holds a bachelor of science in physiological psychology and a masters in sociology from the University of Pittsburgh. She completed her doctorate in science studies at the University of Chicago followed by a master's degree in public health from the Johns Hopkins University as a senior National Cancer Institute postdoctoral fellow in epidemiology. For more information on Dr. Davis, visit www.DevraDavis.org.

Joel Fuhrman, M.D., is a board-certified family physician, bestselling author, and one of the country's leading experts on nutritional medicine. He speaks to audiences at conferences, seminars, and events throughout the United States and Canada. He addresses other physicians at hospital grand rounds and has lectured at benefits for the American Heart Association and the U.S. Olympic Team. Dr. Fuhrman has appeared in hundreds of magazines, on the radio, and on television including: *Good Morning America* (ABC), *The Today Show* (NBC), *Good Day New York* (FOX), The Food Network, CNN, UPN, and the Discovery Channel. His books include: *Eat To Live, Cholesterol Protection for Life,* and *Disease Proof Your Child.* His upcoming book, *Eat for Health,* will be published in January 2008. Dr. Fuhrman teaches nutrition excellence is not only preventative, but is also the most effective therapeutic interventions for most chronic medical conditions. At his Web site, www.DrFuhrman.com, he supplies health and nutrition information and answers people's health and nutrition questions.

Michael Giuliano, M.D., MEd., is director of neonatology at Hackensack University Medical Center and clinical associate professor at SUNY

Downstate, New York. In addition to his clinical responsibilities, he is involved in the entire spectrum of education with college students, medical students, residents, and continuing education. Before coming to Hackensack University Medical Center he was associate director of pediatrics and coordinator for pediatric education at Lenox Hill Hospital. He has been involved in medical education at a national level and as delegate to the Committee on Medical Education to Pediatrics (COMSEP). In his spare time, he's a father to five wonderful children and is an occasional Mets fan.

Mady Hornig, M.D., directs translational research activities at the Center for Infection and Immunity at Columbia University. A physician-scientist board-certified in psychiatry, she is highly regarded for her investigations on brain-immune interactions and their role in the development of autism, attention-deficit/hyperactivity disorder, obsessive-compulsive disorder, and mood disorders.

Named as a College Scholar at Cornell (AB, Biology, Law, and Society, 1978), Dr. Hornig was further educated at The New School for Social Research (MA, Psychology, 1983) and The Medical College of Pennsylvania (M.D., 1988). In 2004, she was the first to show increased risk for neurodevelopmental damage in genetically susceptible mice after early life exposure to subtoxic doses of mercury such as those found in the environment or in biologic products such as vaccines. That same year, she presented at the Institute of Medicine and testified twice before U.S. congressional subcommittees regarding the potential interplay of genetic and temporal factors in creating susceptibility to adverse neurodevelopmental outcomes after infectious or immunotoxic exposures. She is the editor of four books and has published widely on the effects of immune, infectious, and endocrine factors on brain development and function in a wide range of neuropsychiatric conditions.

Dr. Yukiko Kimura is chief of pediatric rheumatology at the Joseph M. Sanzari Children's Hospital of Hackensack University Medical Center. She established the pediatric rheumatology program, the first in New Jersey, in 1991. Today, the program is one of the largest and busiest in the country, with four board-certified pediatric rheumatologists and a multidisciplinary team devoted to improving the lives of children with arthritis and other rheumatic diseases. Dr. Kimura received her M.D. degree from the Albert Einstein College of Medicine. Board-certified in both pediatrics and pediatric rheumatology, she is currently an associate professor of pediatrics at UMDNJ–New Jersey Medical School and a fellow of both the American Academy of Pediatrics and the American College of Rheumatology. She has written many articles and has been invited to lecture nationally and internationally about arthritis in children. She is a coeditor of a new textbook of pediatric rheumatology called *Arthritis in Children and Adolescents.* She was awarded two honors recently by the American College of Rheumatology: a Pediatric Rheumatology Visiting Professorship Award and the Clinician-Scholar-Educator Award.

Philip J. Landrigan, M.D., is a pediatrician who serves as director of the Children's Environmental Health Center, and as chair of the Department of Community and Preventive Medicine at The Mount Sinai School of Medicine in New York City. He's also a professor of pediatrics at Mount Sinai.

Dr. Landrigan obtained his medical degree from the Harvard Medical School in 1967. He has served as a commissioned officer in the United States Public Health Service, and as an Epidemic Intelligence Service Officer and then as a Medical Epidemiologist with the CDC in Atlanta. While at the CDC, Dr. Landrigan served for one year as a field epidemiologist in El Salvador and for another year in northern Nigeria. From 1979 to 1985, he directed the U.S. national program in occupational epidemiology at the National Institute of Occupational Safety and Health in Cincinnati.

Dr. Landrigan is a member of the Institute of Medicine of the National Academy of Sciences, and Editor-in-Chief Emeritus of the American Journal of Industrial Medicine. From 1988 to 1993, Dr. Landrigan chaired a National Academy of Sciences Committee whose final report, Pesticides in the Diets of Infants and Children, and provided the principal intellectual foundation for the Food Quality Protection Act of 1996. He has served on the Presidential Advisory Committee on Gulf War Veteran's Illnesses, and as senior advisor on children's health at the EPA, where he also established a new Office of Children's Health Protection.

Dr. Richard Lathe qualified in Molecular Biology at Edinburgh and Brussels. With a special interest in Neuroscience, he is currently director of Pieta Research in Edinburgh. He was formerly professor at the Universities of Strasbourg and Edinburgh, a codirector of the European Biotechnology College ESBS in Strasbourg, and deputy scientific director at the French company, Transgène. His monograph *Autism, Brain, and Environment* was published last year by Jessica Kingsley Publishers, London and Philadelphia.

Barbara McGoey has been a registered nurse for 24 years. She has been employed in many different areas of nursing; including the pediatric emergency room, pediatric recovery room, orthopedics, pediatric clinic, mother-baby, and regular medical-surgical areas. Prior to coming to Hackensack University Medical Center in 1998, Nurse McGoey worked at Columbia Presbyterian Medical Center in NYC at Babies Hospital. In addition to hospital settings, she has worked as a telephone triage nurse, answering medical questions via the phone when children are home and sick at night. She has also been the nurse coordinator for the medical staff at the Imus Ranch in Ribera, New Mexico, for the past three years. Nurse McGoey received her A.A.S. in Nursing from Kingsborough Community College in Brooklyn, New York, and her B.S.N. from City University State of New York, College of Staten Island.

Mehmet C. Oz, M.D., is professor and vice-chairman of surgery at Columbia University. He directs the Cardiovascular Institute and Complementary Medicine Program at New York Presbyterian Hospital. His research interests include heart replacement surgery, minimally invasive cardiac surgery, complementary medicine, and health care policy. He has authored over 400 original publications, book chapters, and medical books, and has received several patents. He performs over 300 heart operations annually.

Dr. Oz is the health expert on *The Oprah Winfrey Show*. He is chief medical consultant to Discovery Communications and has hosted several shows including *Second Opinion with Dr. Oz* and *Life Line*. His "Transplant!" series on Discovery Health Channel won both a FREDDIE and a Silver TELLY award in September 2006. In addition to numerous appearances on network morning and evening news programs.

Dr. Oz has written three *New York Times* bestsellers: *You: The Owner's Manual, You: The Smart Patient,* and *You: On a Diet,* as well as the award-winning *Healing from the Heart*. He has a regular column in *Esquire* and *Reader's Digest* magazines. He lives in Cliffside Park, New Jersey, with his wife of twenty years, Lisa, and their four children, Daphne, Arabella, Zoe, and Oliver.

Dr. Frederica Perera is professor at Columbia University School of Public Health, where she serves as director of the Columbia Center for Children's Environmental Health. Dr. Perera pioneered the field of molecular epidemiology, conducting the first studies of carcinogen-DNA adducts in human populations and co-editing the principal textbook *Molecular Epidemiology: Principles and Practices*. She has authored over two hundred publications. Her areas of specialization include prevention of environmental risks to children, molecular epidemiology, cancer prevention, environment-susceptibility interactions in cancer, developmental damage, asthma, and risk assessment. Dr. Perera received her undergraduate degree from Harvard University and her masters and doctoral degrees in Public Health from Columbia University. Dr. Perera received the First Irving J. Selikoff Cancer Research Award from The Ramazzini Institute for Occupational and Environmental Health Research in 1995; the Newsweek Club award in 1997;

the First Children's environmental Health Award from The Pew Center for Children's Health and the Environment in 1999; and the Distinguished Lecturer in Occupational and Environmental Cancer at the National Cancer Institute in 2002, and an *Honoris Causa* (Honorary Doctorate) from the Jagiellonian University of Krakow in 2005.

Lawrence D. Rosen, M.D., is a board-certified general pediatrician committed to family-centered, holistic child health care. He practices in northern New Jersey and consults at the Children's Hospital at Hackensack University Medical Center, serving as a medical advisor to the Deirdre Imus Environmental Center. Dr. Rosen is a nationally recognized expert in Pediatric Integrative Medicine, acting as chair of the Integrative Pediatrics Council, a nonprofit foundation dedicated to transforming children's health care. Dr. Rosen is also a founding member of the American Academy of Pediatrics Provisional Section on Complementary, Holistic and Integrative Medicine. He is a frequent speaker at both professional and consumer gatherings, discussing topics such as holistic care of the newborn and the integrative management of autism. Dr. Rosen is a graduate of New York Medical College and the Massachusetts Institute of Technology. He completed his residency and chief residency in pediatrics at Mount Sinai Hospital in New York and is a Fellow of the American Academy of Pediatrics.

Michael Rosenbaum, M.D., is an Associate Program Director of the General Clinical Research Center and Columbia Presbyterian Medical Center. Board-certified in Pediatric Endocrinology, he has a longstanding interest in clinical research relating to alterations of energy expenditure to body weight. He has worked with other experts in a clinical study regarding the role of leptin and body composition. Dr. Rosenbaum has just completed a pilot study designed to examine the effects of supervised exercise and nutritional and health education on metabolic risk factors for type II diabetes mellitus in children. He is working on an NIH/NIDDK-funded grant in human obesity.

Susan Sencer, M.D., is the director of hematology/oncology at Children's of Minnesota. She guides the clinical, research, programming, education, funding, and marketing aspects of integrative medicine for children and families in the hematology/oncology program at Children's Hospitals and Clinics. Dr. Sencer received a bachelor's degree in psychology from Grinnell College and her M.D. from the University of Minnesota School of Medicine, specializing in pediatrics and in hematology/oncology, and continuing adjunct faculty status with the medical school. Dr. Sencer has over twenty years of training and experience in pediatrics, hematology/oncology, and complementary/alternative medicine. In 1998, she was the recipient of a Bush Foundation Physician Mid-Career Fellowship to study the use of complementary and alternative medicine in children with cancer. She lectures locally and nationally on pediatric integrative medicine and is an expert on the uses of herbals and supplements in pediatric oncology.

Kenneth R. Warren, Ph.D., is the Associate Director for Basic Research within the NIH's National Institute on Alcohol Abuse and Alcoholism (NIAAA). Since joining the staff of NIAAA in 1976, he has held a number of institute positions, from scientific review administrator to director of the Office of Scientific Affairs (OSA). During his twenty two years as OSA director, he was also the executive secretary for the National Advisory Council on Alcohol Abuse and Alcoholism.

In February 1977, Dr. Warren organized the first national research workshop on fetal alcohol syndrome (FAS). This conference set a research agenda on FAS and also recommended that NIAAA alert the medical community about FAS and the risks posed by prenatal alcohol. Dr. Warren secured the approval of the then Department of Health Education and Welfare for the issuance of a health advisory, which first appeared in June 1977.

Subsequently, Dr. Warren took the lead in developing a congressional report on the health hazards of alcohol use. Dr. Warren prepared several chapters for the report, including one on *Birth Defects and Anomalies*. One outcome of this 1980 report was the issuance of the Surgeon General's Advisory on Fetal Alcohol Syndrome in May 1981, for which Dr. Warren was the lead contributor. Twenty-four years later, he again played a significant role in the development and issuance of an updated Surgeon General's Advisory in February 2005.

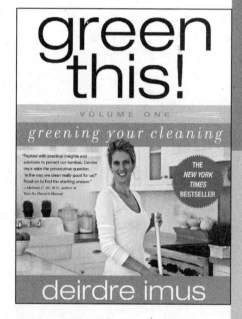